Bircher-Benner Manuals

Enjoy Food without Table Salt
Manual for Curing Salt-Sensitive Hypertension

Dietary instructions
for the prevention and treatment
of diseases caused by too much table salt
with recipes,
detailed advice
and a treatment plan
developed by a medical centre
dedicated to state-of-the-art healing

Dr.med.Andres Bircher
and colleagues of the
Bircher-Benner Medical Centre
Lilli Bircher, Pascal Bircher and
Anne-Cécile Bircher

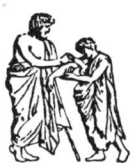

EDITION BIRCHER-BENNER
CH-8784 BRAUNWALD

Bircher-Benner Manuals

1. Manual for patients suffering from multiple sclerosis, Parkinson's disease and other neurodegenerative diseases
2. Manual for patients with liver and gallbladder conditions
3. Manual for families and children
4. Manual for fresh juices, raw vegetables and fruit dishes
5. Manual for improvement of the immune system and against susceptibility to infections
6. Manual for mountaineers and athletes
7. Manual for diabetics
8. Manual for support and preventive therapy for lung diseases
9. Enjoy food without table salt
10. Manual for patients with rheumatism and arthritis
11. Manual for men with prostate conditions
12. Manual for patients with kidney and bladder conditions
13. Manual for venous diseases
14. Manual for patients with gastrointestinal conditions
15. Manual for nutrition during pregnancy and lactation
16. Manual for gynaecological problems and menopause
17. Manual for prevention of cancer and accompanying therapies
18. Manual for patients suffering from headaches and migraines
19. Manual for patients with hypertension, cardiovascular disease and arteriosclerosis
20. Manual for overcoming anxiety and depression
21. Manual for patients with skin diseases or sensitive skin
22. Manual for persons suffering from stress
23. Manual for persons suffering from allergies
24. Manual for prevention of dementia and Alzheimer's disease
25. Manual for internal treatment of eye problems
26. Healthy and slim, manual for treatment of weight problems, overweight and anorexia

These manuals are the result of global research, of the development of the art and science of medicine over more than a century, and of the experience of the renowned Bircher-Benner Medical Centre. The reader will benefit from the helpful support of the well-informed physician every step of the way.

5th edition 2020. Translated from the original German

All rights reserved, including the right of reproduction in excerpts, photomechanical reproduction and translation

info@bircher-benner.com   www.bircher-benner.com

Book orders: edition@bircher-benner.com
© Copyright by Edition Bircher-Benner, CH 8784 Braunwald
® The trademarks Bircher and Bircher-Benner are protected worldwide
Printed in Germany

While the suggestions in this book have been carefully reviewed by the authors and the publisher, they cannot be guaranteed. The authors and the publisher hereby disclaim all liability for personal injury, property damage and any type of financial loss.

Typesetting: Eberl & Koesel Studio, Altusried-Krugzell
Printing and binding: Pustet, Regensburg

Table of Contents

Preface 5

Blood Pressure Regulation in the Kidney 8
    The Renin-Angiotensin-Aldosterone System of Blood Pressure Regulation . . 8

Salt-Sensitive Hypertension 10
    Osmotic Storage of Salt in Tissues 10
    Effect of Salt Storage on Blood Vessels and Blood Pressure 10
    Effect of a Low-Salt Diet on Blood Pressure 11
    Epigenetic Inheritance of Salt Sensitivity 11
    Effect of Table Salt Storage on the Blood Vessels 11
    Effects of Salinisation and Saccharisation (Glycation) of the Inner Layer of the Blood Vessels 12

Oxidative Stress at the Centre of the Causes of Degenerative Diseases and Dementia 14

The Problem of Food Energy 17

Order Therapy for Hypertension 18
    Basics for Understanding the Causes and Nutritional Treatment of Hypertension 18
    Two Kinds of Food Energy 18
    Photon Storage in Living Tissues 18
    The Basic Regulation System of the Soft Connective Tissue 19
    The Meaning of Food Economy 20
    The Integral Law of Nutrition 22
    Vibrancy of Food 22

Principles of the Bircher-Benner Diet and Order Therapy 23

Order of Life and Physical Exercise 25

Menus for the Low-Salt Diet, for Patients with Hypertension and Heart Problems	26
Week Plan for Strict Salt-free, Natrium-low Diet	26
Menu for 1 Week of Salt-free Diet (Milder Form)	27
Recipes for Salt-free and Low-salt Food	29
Juices	29
Gruel Added to Juices	30
Bircher Muesli	30
Raw Vegetables and Salads	32
Salad Dressings	33
Suggestions for Dressings to go with Salads and Raw Vegetables	36
Milk Types	37
Butter, Vegetable Fats and Oils	38
Gentle Cooking and Steaming	39
Soups	39
Soup Additions	40
Vegetables	43
Salads of Cooked Vegetables	50
Potato Dishes	51
Grain Dishes	54
Sauces	58
Sandwiches	61
Desserts	62
Healthy Teas	67
Table Regarding Glycaemic Index and Glycaemic Charge	69
List of Recipes	73
Notes	77
Index	80

Preface

Table salt has always been one of the most popular stimulants. In the Celtic-Germanic region, the production of sea salt was on a large scale as early as the Bronze Age[1]. The Sumerians preserved their food with salt. Pliny the Elder and Lucius Columella estimated that daily salt consumption in ancient Rome corresponded to 25 g/person. Through the 19th century, table salt was used mainly as a preservative for meat, cabbage and beans[2].

Yet few people are aware of the damage caused by excessive amounts of table salt. In the 1970s, high salt consumption was recognised as a major cause of hypertension, and consequently a significant source of cardiovascular disease. The Food and Drug Administration has estimated consumption of table salt in the US at 8.4 g/person, which corresponds to about 2¼ teaspoons per day. US authorities have issued guidelines to reduce table salt in all convenience foods, as they account for 75 % of salt consumption. They estimate that a 40 % reduction could save 500,000 lives in the course of the next decade. The daily human salt demand depends on the climate and season. Today it is estimated to be in the range of 1.8–6.4 g per day. The World Health Organisation currently recommends 5 g per day, or about 1.2 level teaspoons.

Many people underestimate their salt consumption, as three-quarters of it comes from convenience foods and only about one-quarter from salting. Cured convenience foods such as fish, meat and sausage products are popular. Pickling salt is table salt with the addition of 0.4–0.5 % sodium nitrite. Nitrite combines the radical nitric oxide (NO) with myoglobin into heat-stable nitrosomyoglobin, which gives cured meat a more appetising, stable red colour. As a result, all products cured with nitrite are carcinogenic.

There is also the sodium content from sodium fluoride. Since 2006, sodium fluoride has been added to table salt throughout the EU to prevent tooth decay. Eighty percent of the population uses sodium fluoride. The addition of spices and other flavourings, such as glutamate, leads to the extensive range of seasoning salts. Spices are supposed to flavour the salt, while salt has a stabilising effect on the spices.

The processes that lead to hypertension are complex. Some influences are genetic and environmental, though it is not clear why people are not equally sensitive to high levels of table salt. In about 70 % of the population, even a relatively small overdose of table salt causes hypertension ("salt-sensitive hypertension"). Others have a higher toleration for table salt, even storing excessive salt in their body tissues. However, high salt concentrations also have pathogenic effects on the vascular system, independent of blood pressure in people in whom the high salt concentrations do not immediately produce hypertension. An excessive amount of table salt damages the inner layer of the blood vessels and the endothelium, and also causes arteriosclerosis.

The concealed consumption of salt in industrial convenience products and fast food has increased drastically. At the same time, we see a massive increase in hypertension. Thirty percent of the world's population suffers from hypertension today. More than half of all adults over the age of 19 in industrialised countries suffer from hypertension and take antihypertensive medication. Given such statistics, the "average adult" has hypertension. It is no longer "the norm" not to have hypertension and not to have to take antihypertensive medication.

Table salt is not the only thing that causes hypertension. The high consumption of white flour products and sugar also damages the inner layer of the vessels through direct chemical reaction of the sugars with the endothelium. This innermost layer regulates the anatomical structure and muscle tension throughout the vascular wall. The damage caused by this excess of table salt and sugar destroys the endothelium's ability to regulate the muscle tension of the blood vessels and their structure and fibre content. This is referred to as endothelial dysfunction. The vessels narrow and can no longer be widened when blood flow increases, initially increasing blood pressure at exertion or excitement (labile hypertension). Then the vessel walls harden due to the storage of hard connective tissue (collagen). This causes constantly elevated blood pressure, even during relaxation and sleep (fixed hypertension). Metabolic waste products then become increasingly deposited in the intercellular substance (matrix) of the vessel walls. This leads to inflammation and thickening the vessel walls into arteriosclerotic plaques, until they begin to store cholesterol and calcium. High consumption of salt, white flour and sugar thereby produces arteriosclerosis at a young age.

Angina pectoris and myocardial infarction develop if this occurs in the coronary arteries; in the carotid arteries that supply the brain, it leads to cerebral apoplexy. In arteries of the legs, intermittent claudication (claudicatio intermittens) leads to cramps and pain when walking, since the leg arteries are narrowed by arteriosclerosis and can no longer supply the blood and oxygen needed.

High consumption of salt, white flour and sugar will damage the fine vessels of the kidneys and the eyes, and prevents the aqueous humour of the eyes from draining through the fine structures in the corner of the eye, which in turn increases pressure in the eyes. This leads to glaucoma, blindness due to glaucoma, and macular degeneration.

All of these tragic diseases seem to be a tragic fate. In fact, they have nothing to do with "fate", since they can be reliably prevented by following a diet of living vegetarian whole foods with a high proportion of raw vegetables seasoned with fresh herbs, while avoiding all irritants such as excessive amounts of table salt, sugar, coffee and alcohol. While these diseases cannot be prevented by any drug, they can be prevented by a diet and lifestyle that meet our biological needs.

A low-salt diet is necessary if hypertension has already developed or if cardiovascular disease has progressed. The recipes given in this book were developed in the famous Bircher-Benner Klinik. Creating low-salt and salt-free recipes that are not bland but delicious is a fine art. This manual is based on vast experience in the treatment of people suffering from nutrition-related diseases. Since Dr. med. Maximilian Bircher-Benner discovered the immense healing effect of a strict, fresh, plant-based diet and an orderly lifestyle more than a century ago, the Bircher-Benner Klinik, today called the Bircher-

Benner Medical Centre, has healed thousands of people suffering from the "diseases of civilisation" that today are spreading massively. This manual describes one of the building blocks for therapy that does not merely suppress symptoms, but tackles the root causes of disease in order to cure it. The recipes can be used in practice. For the physician, this book is a great time saver in counselling patients.

Dr. med. Andres Bircher

Blood Pressure Regulation in the Kidney

Twenty percent of the blood flow of the circulatory system goes to the kidneys, which perform enormous filtration and reabsorption functions. These permit the elimination of water-soluble toxins and metabolic waste products.

The Renin-Angiotensin-Aldosterone System of Blood Pressure Regulation

This control cycle of hormones and enzymes regulates the balance of fluid volume in the blood and body. Specialised tissues in the kidneys, called the juxtaglomerular apparatus, produce the renin enzyme, which comprises:

- specialised cells in the smallest arteries (arterioles) that supply the renal corpuscle (vas afferens)
- specialised cells of the urinary tubule that runs near the vas afferens (macula densa)
- specialised cells of the connective tissue (mesangial cells)

This entire juxtaglomerular apparatus measures blood pressure in the vas afferens vessel that leads to the renal tubule and the salt content of the primary urine in the urinary tubule. It also reacts to signals from the autonomic nervous system and to various hormones. The hormone renin is produced in the cells of the vas afferens and stored in fine granules in the cells.

Renin is released into the blood when:

- the kidneys receive less blood
- blood pressure drops significantly
- less primary urine is filtered from the renal corpuscles into the urinary tubule
- the concentration of salt in the urinary tubule decreases
- the sympathetic nervous system is activated (e.g. excitement, fear, anger, effort)

Blood contains angiotensin, which is produced by the liver. Renin splits off angiotensin I, which in turn is converted into angiotensin II by an enzyme (angiotensin converting enzyme, ACE) that constricts the blood vessels in the entire circulation. This raises the blood pressure. Angiotensin II in the adrenal cortex also releases the aldosterone hormone. This acts on the renal tubules, causing them to reabsorb much more salt and water back into the circulation. Consequently blood volume increases and blood pressure rises even more.

However, angiotensin II also acts on the pituitary gland, causing it to secrete a hormone that forces the kidney to reabsorb even more water into the circulation; this hormone of the posterior lobe of the pituitary gland is therefore called antidiuretic hormone, ADH. Blood pressure increases when more water enters the circulation.

In the brain, these hormones increase thirst and cravings for salt.
High blood pressure means that the angiotensin II hormones and aldosterone

inhibit the release of renin to keep the entire system from being overactivated (negative feedback).

This entire hormonal cascade provides vital protection to stabilise blood pressure and blood volume, and to prevent dehydration.

Too much table salt in the diet renders the kidneys unable to remove the excess salt from the urine, causing it to accumulate in the body and drawing water with it[3,4]. The system regulating blood pressure is then overstrained and unable to maintain blood pressure in the normal range. Many hypertension drugs act on enzymes in this cascade, in order to lower blood levels of angiotensin II and aldosterone. This short-term fix-it does not address the cause of hypertension, so more and more drugs have to be prescribed for it. See Bircher-Benner Manual No. 19 for patients with hypertension, cardiovascular disease and arteriosclerosis.

Salt-Sensitive Hypertension

There is a general, long-accepted theory that an excess of table salt produces hypertension, because more salt is ingested from the food than the kidneys can excrete. The salt accumulates in the intercellular space and draws water with it by osmotic means, so that a general flooding of the tissues produces hypertension.

Osmotic Storage of Salt in Tissues

However, recent findings have shown that the stored salt not only spreads in the extracellular space, but also goes beyond the extracellular space and blood volume. Negatively charged macromolecules of the subcutaneous tissue chemically bind sodium and chloride ions of the table salt, rendering the table salt osmotically inactive so that it will not draw any water.

The amount of osmotically stored table salt causes an invasion of immune cells, monocytes, and macrophages (phagocytes). These produce a protein called tonicity response element binding protein (TonEBP) and a substance (vascular endothelial growth factor C) that stimulates the formation of new vessels. This leads to intensive formation of new lymphatic vessels (lymphangiogenesis). Many new lymphatic vessels are formed and the lymphatic drainage system is expanded in order to bring the excess table salt back into the bloodstream. Table salt draws water in the bloodstream, increasing the blood volume and raising the blood pressure.

Effect of Salt Storage on Blood Vessels and Blood Pressure

Table salt is stored osmotically ineffectively in the skin, intestines and endothelium of blood vessels. The innermost cell layer of the blood vessels, the endothelium, produces a layer also referred to as the capsule or mucous membrane, and is called the glycocalyx. It consists of multiple sugars (polysaccharides) that are chemically (i.e. covalently) bound to the proteins of the cell membrane, the protein sugar molecules (glycoproteids) and the fatty substances of the cell membrane (membrane lipids, glycolipids, phospholipids, cholesterol and sphingolipids). They cover the innermost layer of the endothelium of the blood vessels. This sensitive, complex glycocalyx of the blood vessels is damaged both by table salt and by high blood sugar levels. As a result, the cells of the endothelium are damaged. They are rendered unable to correctly control the structure and muscle tension of the blood vessels, so that the blood vessels become narrow, store hard connective tissue and become increasingly hardened. This is called endothelial dysfunction.

Narrow, hardened blood vessels cause the vascular resistance to gradually increase, which can be seen in the rise of the lower (diastolic) blood pressure value. Now the blood pressure remains constantly elevated even in sleep and relaxation (fixed hypertension).
Not all people are equally sensitive to table salt. When blood pressure rises by more than 10 % as a result of several

high-salt meals, this is called salt-sensitive hypertension.

About 1 g/day of table salt (NaCl) is necessary for life. Studies in animals, as well as epidemiological and clinical studies, demonstrate the direct link between high salt consumption, hypertension and vascular-circulatory diseases[5,6,7,8,9,10,11,12,13,14,15]. Many epidemiological studies have demonstrated that excessive salt consumption is associated with an increased risk of cardiovascular disease[16,17,18,19]. It has also been shown that the blood pressure response to high salt consumption varies greatly from person to person[20,21,22]. Increased salt consumption also contributes to the development of overweight and obesity[23]. Experimental research and studies in humans have so far not rendered any fully conclusive explanation for the pathophysiological processes leading to hypertension.

Effect of a Low-Salt Diet on Blood Pressure

In comparative studies, a short-term low-salt diet does not lower previously normal blood pressure in all subjects, but it does in 26 % of subjects. Fifty-one percent of patients with elevated blood pressure respond to a relatively short-term low-salt diet. The blood level of the renin hormone does not change significantly, but the blood volume does[24]. However, a long-term low-salt diet is an effective contribution to antihypertensive therapy in all people. Several prospective cohort studies have demonstrated that cardiovascular disease, myocardial infarction, stroke, and death are highly clustered in people who are sensitive to table salt[25,26].

Women are slightly more sensitive to table salt than men. Sensitivity generally increases with age, especially where blood pressure was already slightly elevated to begin with. Plant-based foods are rich in potassium. A diet high in potassium from plants and low in sodium is shown to be particularly effective against hypertension in short-term, repeated and long-term trials[27,28].

Epigenetic Inheritance of Salt Sensitivity

There has been a thorough search for genetic causes of salt sensitivity. Several gene mutations were found that affect the strength of salt excretion in the renal tubules and were associated with hypertension[29]. These are single gene defects. Nine years later, it was recognised that epigenetic changes, rather than genetic mutations, were affecting salt-sensitive people. These are hereditary genetic changes that affect blood pressure without any alteration to the genetic material. They are heritable changes in the activity of genes, without any change in the gene itself[30]. Modern genetic research increasingly discovered the great relevance of heredity through epigenetic changes. This is caused by environmental influences, the type of diet and lifestyle. Soon thereafter, it was shown that table salt is stored in the glucosamine molecules of the intercellular substance without drawing water after it[31,32].

Effect of Table Salt Storage on the Blood Vessels

Sodium storage in the intercellular substance causes infiltration of the intercellular space with phagocytes (macrophages)[33]. These macrophages secrete the endothelial vascular growth factor (VEGF), triggering a strong formation of new lymphatic vessels and increasing production of nitric oxide (NO) by the endothelium of the blood vessels. These findings have greatly changed the scientific understanding of saline storage[34].

The surface layer inside the blood vessels is another important salt barrier and a place of salt storage without osmotic effect. This inner layer is negatively charged. High salt consumption causes sodium to chemically bind to this layer[35,36] and damages the inner layer of blood vessels; it constricts them by reducing nitric oxide production in the endothelium, and stiffens the vessels[37]. This serves as evidence of damage to the vessels; their constriction and hardening through structural remodelling due to high salt consumption has been scientifically proven in this way[38,39].

High consumption of salt thus damages both the blood vessels and the kidneys. A low-salt diet essentially contributes to curing hypertension and preventing cardiovascular disease and arteriosclerosis, preventing heart attack, stroke and other health disasters.

Endothelial dysfunction and arteriosclerosis
Endothelial dysfunction results from damage to the inner walls of blood vessels, as previously discussed, due to chemical storage of sodium in high-salt diets; and from glucose in frequent high blood glucose levels. For a long time, the inner skin of the blood vessels was considered a purely mechanical protective layer and seal. Thanks to more specific research, it is now known that the endothelium of the vessels regulates the muscle tension (tone) of the vascular wall, and thus the width and elasticity of the vessels. The innermost cell layer (endothelium) also suppresses the migration of muscle cells and binds immune cells (adhesion of the monocytes), activates them to form inflammatory mediators, and controls their migration from the blood vessels into the intercellular substance and the tissues.

The endothelium influences the substance exchange between the blood and intercellular liquids (homoeostasis), and also influences coagulation of the blood and the ability of dissolving clots again (fibrinolysis).

In healthy people, the endothelium of the vessels regulates the vascular resistance as follows:

As a result of an oxygen deficit, strong flowing shear forces and/or the effect of the neurovegetative transfer substance acetylcholine, the endothelium cells produce nitrogen monoxide (NO), which has a severely laxative effect on the muscle cells. It penetrates the vascular walls to the smooth muscle cells of the vascular walls and causes them to go slack, and hence, expand. As a result, the vascular resistance diminishes (vasodilatation), causing more blood to flow through the respective vessel.

Diabetics suffer from endothelial dysfunction. This means that the regulation capacity of the blood vessels is reduced by a number of impairments in the formation of nitrogen monoxide (NO), so that they cannot go slack. This raises the blood pressure.

Effects of Salinisation and Saccharisation (Glycation) of the Inner Layer of the Blood Vessels

The phenomenon of salinisation and glycation and endothelial dysfunction take place in every person who consumers a high amount of table salt, white flour and sugary food. It is one of the most important causes of the widespread disease of arteriosclerosis. Diabetes mellitus is feared for its vascular complications. They occur 2–4 times more frequently than in people without diabetes. Increased blood sugar levels (hyperglycaemia) lead to formation of diacylglycerol. This molecule and, as has been shown, the binding of sodium to the inner layer of the blood vessels activates the enzyme protein kinase C (PK-C), which suppresses the formation of nitrogen monoxide (NO) so that the vascular endothelium cannot regulate vessel width anymore. This enzyme (PK-C) also stimulates formation of the substance endothelin-1 (ET-1), which constricts the blood vessels (vasoconstriction). This narrows the vessels and increases the vascular resistance, so that the blood pressure rises and circulation of the organs reduces noticeably.

The same enzyme (PK-C) also activates the enzyme NADP-oxydase, which forms reactive oxidising substances and free radicals (reactive oxygen species, ROS). It is therefore involved in the creation of oxidative stress that is described in detail below. These very strongly oxidising ROS react with the nitrogen monoxide formed at the same time (NO) and convert it to peroxinitrite ($ONOO^-$).

Peroxinitrite is a dangerous, extremely oxidising radical. It causes an entire series of oxidising processes and hardens the connective tissue of the vascular walls by the storage of collagen fibres, fibronectin and laminin.

The insulin level, which is at least initially increased in type-II diabetes, and the insulin resistance are also relevant for hardening of the vascular walls and their inability to expand. This leads to a partial interference with the insulin signal path at the cells of the vascular inner walls (endothelium) and further reduces their ability to form nitrogen monoxide (NO). In addition, the insulin resistance promotes the formation of substances that drive arteriosclerosis (plasminogen activator 1 [PA-1] and ET-1, etc.).

The abundant fatty tissue leads to increased inflammation readiness in overweight people, since it excretes adipokines. These specifically include the tumour necrosis factor α (TNF-α). This is involved both in the development of insulin resistance and in reduction of the regulation capacity of the blood vessels, exacerbated by the damage caused by sodium deposits at high salt consumption (endothelial dysfunction)[40]. Hardening of the vascular walls leads to fixed hypertension. This means that it can no longer drop in sleep and at rest, due to the narrowing and stiffness of the vessels.

Oxidative Stress at the Centre of the Causes of Degenerative Diseases and Dementia

Oxidative stress is at the centre of the causes of degenerative diseases and dementia.

The following cause the organism to suffer oxidative stress: unsuitable nutrition; stimulants; environmental stress; a disorderly lifestyle; ionising, UV-A and electromagnetic radiation; frequently high blood sugar levels, as we have already seen, and glycation and salination of the tissues. This leads to a metabolic situation in which a quantity of reactive oxygen species ROS (reactive oxygen species) is produced that exceeds physiological levels. These highly reactive oxidising substances are molecules with at least one unsaturated electron pair, which makes them particularly reactive. They are produced in the mitochondria, the "power plants" of the cells, that break down glucose through electron transfer and the enzyme cytochrome P 450-oxidase. This produces the superoxide anion radical (O_2-), hydrogen superoxide (H_2O_2), the hydroxide radical ($OH*$) and nitric oxide ($NO*$).

Healthy cells can neutralise these highly reactive oxygen compounds by providing neutralising substances. The most important anti-oxidative substance provided by the body is glutathione, a peptide that it produces from the three amino acids: glutamic acid, cysteine and glycine. Other important antioxidants are ubiquinone (activated coenzyme Q 10), vitamins C and E, selenium and many bioactive secondary plant substances from plant-based food.

In the case of oxidative stress in the metabolism, these reserves have been depleted. Oxidised glutathione can no longer be sufficiently returned to its active, reduced form, since the enzyme glutathione reductase is depleted, as are other detoxification enzymes such as peroxide dismutase and catalase. The highly reactive oxidants (ROS) thus remain in the metabolism, where they can damage large molecules (macro molecules) both inside and outside the cells.

This has dangerous consequences. The unsaturated fatty acids of the cell membranes are oxidised (lipid peroxidation), causing the destruction of the mitochondria, exhausting the cells and requiring them to expend considerably more energy to maintain their electrical membrane potentials. Moreover, lipid peroxidation damages the lipid-containing myelin sheaths of the fast-conducting nerve fibres in the brain and the spinal cord, and in the nerves outside the central nervous system. There will be further damage to proteins (protein peroxidation) and to hereditary peroxidation (DNA peroxidation), which causes the DNA molecules of the hereditary material to split (genetic mutation) and may lead to the conversion of healthy cells into tumour or cancer cells.

Oxidative stress means that the organism is in a premature aging process that will severely reduce life expectancy. Glucose metabolism (in the respiratory chain of the mitochondria) produces water as its end product when in heals. In about 2 % of cases, errors occur so that, for example, an oxygen atom will connect to one instead of two hydrogen atoms, systematically creating a highly reactive fission product of water, the hydroxyl radical (OH*). This free radical is highly reactive because the oxygen atom of the OH* radical is actively searching for an additional electron from any other molecule. Other radicals include the nitrogen oxide radical (NO*), the chloride radical (Cl*) and the bromine radical (Br*).

The importance of free radicals is currently the object of much scientific interest in connection with research into the causes of various degenerative diseases, specifically neurodegenerative diseases such as Alzheimer's disease (AD), multiple sclerosis (MS), amyotrophic lateral sclerosis, Huntington's disease, Parkinson's disease and diabetic neuropathy. Many studies suggest that destruction of the brain stem ganglions by free radicals is a cause of these increasingly common diseases. Multiple sclerosis shows indications of damage to the myelin sheaths from free radicals, so that the immune system reacts against the oxidised lipids. The same happens in diabetic neuropathy.

Scientists today accept that oxidative stress is one of the key causes of neurodegenerative diseases. The process begins with the oxidation of proteins and enzymes, whose spatial structure (tertiary structure) consequently changes and forms an insoluble beta folding sheet structure that is then deposited in the form of aggregates, the Lewy bodies in Parkinson's disease; or β-amyloid plaques and now-insoluble TAU proteins in Alzheimer's disease, in the brain, where it destroys the nerve cells.

Usually the correct folding of the protein is achieved by means of special protein complexes (chaperons). It is suspected that these chaperone complexes are changed by oxidative and nitrosative stress, so that they can no longer perform their function in the production of a correct three-dimensional structure of the proteins. The insoluble degenerative proteins deposited inside and outside the nerve cells cause programmed cell death (apoptosis). Cell death is caused by excessive excretion of the activating neurotransmitter glutamate . Glutamate activates a receptor in the cell membranes (NMDA receptor) that triggers a permanent calcium flow into the nerve cells. This activates an enzyme (NO-synthase), which causes the nitric oxide radical (NO*) to form. In the mitochondria, excess calcium inhibits cell respiration, causing massive formation of free radicals (ROS). The radical NO* is further oxidised into the highly reactive peroxynitrite, which together with the other free radicals (ROS) massively damages the membranes by lipid peroxidation. This damage releases cytochrome C, which triggers the biologically specified cascade of cell destruction (apoptosis). The brain has a cell-preserving substance that protects the nerve cells from destruction by apoptosis. Thus they would be protected by healthy adjacent cells. However, since the adjacent cells are also attacked, this protection factor is absent and cell death spreads throughout the brain tissue.

Bircher-Benner Manual No. 24 for the prevention of dementia and Alzheimer's disease will inform you in more detail about the causes of dementia. Manual No. 1 for patients with multiple sclerosis, Parkinson's disease and other neurodegenerative diseases explains the causes, prevention and, to the extent possible, the healing of these neurodegenerative diseases.

Oxidative stress contributes to the damage to the inner layer of blood vessels caused by high levels of salt and sugar. A diet rich in antioxidant phytochemicals counteracts this destruction. Bircher-Benner Manual No. 4 for fresh juices, raw vegetables and fruit dishes provides detailed information on this, including tables for the choice of suitable foods.

The Problem of Food Energy

Officially recognised dietary recommendations are based on an understanding of food energy in the form of pure heat energy (calories), and thus the *first law of thermodynamics*, formulated in 1842 by German doctor Julius Robert Mayer. It was the basis for formulation of the law on preservation of energy by Hermann von Helmholz in 1847, and states that calorific energy is never lost in a closed system during mechanical or chemical processes (i.e. it is always preserved). In 1865, German physicist Rudolf Clausius found the contradiction between the first law of thermodynamics and reality, and formulated the *second law of thermodynamics*, stating that the thermal energy in a closed system may not be lost, but that physical disorder occurs in any spontaneous chemical or mechanical process. He called this entropy and thus proved that the perpetuum mobile (a motor running without energy supply) is not possible.

Clausius marked the beginning of a new understanding of the quality of energies. These findings were included in the sciences of chemistry and physics, but surprisingly never in medicine and nutrition. Maximilian Bircher-Benner corrected this in his teachings on food, published in Berlin in 1905. He applied the second law of thermodynamics to food energy[41,42]. Living foods made of plants that have photosynthesis were assigned the highest available food energy (see "Two kinds of food energy" below).

Bircher-Benner's understanding of food energy according to its qualitative value has been confirmed in all respects by recent research in biophysics, biophoton research and molecular biology[43,44,45,46,47,48,49].

The biophysical quality and order of foods forms the basis of the nutritional science underlying this manual. The surprising deficit in the current medical paradigm concerning these findings is the reason why permanent healing of obesity and type 2 diabetes mellitus is usually impossible in accordance with the widespread methodology. Results are quite different when the Bircher-Benner diet described in this manual is adhered to.

Order Therapy for Hypertension

Basics for Understanding the Causes and Nutritional Treatment of Hypertension

Two Kinds of Food Energy

Physicists have identified two types of energy: orderly and chaotic. Orderly energy saves information. Chaotic energy cannot save anything. Heat energy (calories) (is chaotic energy. Sunlight is the most highly ordered form of energy. Its complex information content is like a large symphony. Listening to a symphony does not produce heat, but it provides information; it is a highly orderly sound structure that triggers precise sensations and feelings. With its complex oscillations, sunlight conveys and orders the genetically specified information that is needed for growth, differentiation and regeneration of all life on earth.

Photon Storage in Living Tissues

One green leaf contains about a hundred thousand chlorophyll funnels. At the base of each funnel, there are two chlorophyll A-molecules. The funnel reflects the incoming light into the base, where the two chlorophyll A-molecules enter a maximum resonance, synchronised with the oscillations of the solar radiation. Physicists call this "coherence", in which the waves of sunlight become standing light waves called photons. Their energy, and therefore the information and resonance from sunlight, flows through the entire plant body, all the way down to the roots. Only a little of it is emitted as UV light, and it is invisible to the human eye.

All living cells store UV light in their molecules, particularly in the ring-shaped (aromatic) molecules. The double helix of the genetic material in the cell cores of deoxyribonucleic acid (DNA) stores most light by far. The double helix can coil to the right or left and can form protrusions shaped like clover leaves, radiating specific UV light spectrums. The wound double helix of the DNA serves as a cavity resonator for the rhythmic amplification of UV light in vital cells. Amplification takes place rhythmically according to the laser principle. For a laser to begin functioning, it must receive a certain basic amount of energy. Physicists call this minimally necessary energy the "laser threshold". In their experiments, researchers of the International Academy for Biophoton Research measured the laser threshold in plant-based cell tissues[43].

Just like plants, human and animal cells are forms made up of light while they are alive. This is the difference between life and death. They also store light as UV light in their genetic material deoxyribonucleic acid (DNA)[40]. We lack the ability to photosynthesise, however, and direct application of sunlight to the skin is far from enough to keep our light storage above the laser threshold.

Plant cells store the photons from sunlight in incredible amounts. It could be shown that ultra-weak cell radiation[41] is nothing but radiation leakage, a tiny leak of UV light through the cell membrane.

Measurements showed that laser amplification of the light is 10^4 times stronger in DNA than that provided by the best technical laser devices. The inside of cells therefore represents an extraordinary light space.

Our photon storage must be fed daily with a sufficient amount of vital photon-containing foods, i.e. fresh plant-based raw foods.

The transmission of the information of the vital foods from photosynthesis to our organism takes place by information transfer, or through coherence, just as during photosynthesis. This means that our own sensation of life, life energy and life information is renewed and reordered again and again in the roughly 50 trillion cells of our body by entering into a shared resonance with the oscillation patterns and complex information of sunlight when the photons are transferred.

In terms of energy, the cell's interior differs fundamentally from inanimate nature. Biophysicists call the inside of the cell a dissipative system, which is an ordered structure found in systems that are formed far from thermodynamic equilibrium. Russian-Belgian researcher Ilya Prigogine received a Nobel prize for his work on this subject.

Intense photon storage removes the energy inside the cell so far from the thermodynamic balance that the second law of thermodynamics no longer applies. Thus the principle of chaos, which is valid outside all living things, becomes an ordering principle. Prigogine called this the coherence principle[49].

When living foods are missing from our nutrition, the photon content in our cells declines. The light content falls until it drops below the laser threshold. The cells partially revert from the principle of order (Prigogine's coherence principle) to the chaos principle of thermodynamics, and then they degenerate.

We consider disease to be a loss of order, i.e. a loss of ordered information. The programme of life enters into disorder, and the lack of living nutrition makes reordering impossible. Many experiments, conducted at the University of Novosibirsk and elsewhere[50,51,52] show that the complex processes of biochemistry in our cells are controlled by information. If there is a lack of living nutrition, this information provided by the genes in the DNA will no longer be continually renewed and ordered. Consequently, the complex biochemical processes of our cells will be thrown into disarray. This is why living raw plant food is important for its energy: it renews and strengthens the ordering resonance in the biological system.

The Basic Regulation System of the Soft Connective Tissue

All cells of the body's organs are embedded in the intercellular substance of the soft connective tissue that runs through all organs and structures. It consists of a dense molecular network (matrix) of sugar-protein molecules called proteoglycans, and is soaked with a rich liquid (interstitial fluid). The soft connective tissue contains spindle-shaped cells that form the network of the intercellular substance and continually adjust it as needed. The blood capillaries run through this intercellular substance with their network, including the nerve endings of the vegetative nervous system. Outside the brain and spinal cord, the capillaries deliberately leak, allowing the nutrients and hormones from the blood to leave the capillaries and enter the intercellular substances. They reach the cells through the molecular network, serving as a molecular sieve.

At the same time, it is our system for conducting and storing biological information – the information of our living organism. There is no direct contact between the blood capillaries and the cells in our bodies, where they penetrate the intercellular substance and loop to the discharging veins there. The intercellular substance is drained by the complex system of lymph vessels and cleansed in the lymph nodes. It is then returned to the venous blood as purified lymph through the large lymph vessels. The nerves have blind ends in the intercellular substance. All information from the nervous system to the cells, and from the cells to the nervous system, is routed through the proteoglycans molecular network. As a result, every piece of information is disseminated throughout the entire body, i.e. the system always reacts as a whole (acupuncture makes use of this). This complex system is our "basic regulation system"[53]. All cells in our bodies are supplied with biological information, hormones, nutrients and oxygen through the intercellular substance and the network of proteoglycan molecules. We have seen how excess table salt is stored in the glucosamine molecules of the intercellular substance. This impairs their function as a molecular sieve, as well as the transport and storage of biological information.

The Meaning of Food Economy[54]

Food economy means that the composition of food must correspond exactly to our biological needs, so that neither too much nor too little is supplied. The body needs very little food, but its composition must be adapted to the biological need as precisely as possible. Our biological system cannot cope with an excess of senselessly supplied nutrients. Such excess produces all the "civilisation diseases" whose subjects fill our hospitals and medical practices

Food economy and food energy are decisive in keeping the complex intercellular substance and our basic regulation system healthy, both in the body and in the central nervous system beyond the blood-brain barrier. Senselessly and excessively supplied nutrients and toxins from a diseased, overloaded, over-acidified metabolism and a sick environment in the stomach and intestines cannot be managed or excreted. They remain in the complex system of the intercellular substance as degenerative metabolic slags. There they gradually hinder the vital exchange of substances, gases, and the storage and flow of biological information. The intercellular substance (also called matrix) is where the entire morbidity of "civilised man" – the civilisation diseases – develops.

The system of basic regulation also includes the environment inside the intestine, with its huge ecosystem of intestinal flora. We have seen that autoimmune processes from an ill milieu in the intestine and a degenerated intestinal flora are encouraged because the immune cells can only acquire defective immune competence under such conditions to be able to distinguish properly between external and internal – between the useful and the harmful.

A diseased environment in the intestine is a huge interference field that strongly impairs the basic regulation of the whole organism. Rot (putrefaction) toxins formed by anaerobic bacteria reach the liver through the oral vein system, and together with nutrients supplied uselessly they overload it considerably. They also slag down its intercellular substance until the innermost liver cells of the liver lobules decay and are replaced by fat cells. This is how fatty liver develops. Anything that it cannot detoxify and make water-soluble goes back into the intestine via the bile ducts. From there it is returned over and over to the liver, which tries to detoxify the matter. Thus rot (putrefaction) toxins, excessive nutrients and metabolic slags continue to circulate between the intestine and the liver (enterohepatic circulation), thereby overloading it. Haemorrhoids are caused by overloading of the veins of the rectum, as they are connected to the portal vein system.

In addition, generally widespread malnutrition, with its concomitant excess of protein, fat and sugars in the metabolism, produces huge amounts of organic acids, strongly oxidising ketonic acids and other ROS (reactive oxygen species). (See the chapter on oxidative stress and its consequences.)

These hugely overtax our anti-oxidative systems. Oxidation means degeneration. Proteins altered by oxidation become insoluble and are deposited as amyloids throughout the body in the intercellular substance. They oxidise the cholesterol, which is protected by unsaturated fatty acids inside the LDL molecule on its transport to the cell membranes in the blood. Oxidation makes it insoluble. It accumulates in the arteries and heart in places of rapid blood flow (fatty streaks). Arteriosclerosis starts to develop at a young age today as a result. Storage of amyloids and other metabolic waste products in the intercellular substance of the arterial walls results in arteriosclerotic plaques, leading to the catastrophe of heart attack or stroke. Equally, varicose veins develop, arthritis forms in the synovial mucosa of the joints, nephrosis occurs in the capillary tangles of the kidneys, and there is even diabetic kidney failure. The fine, connective-tissue structure of the trabecular bones degenerates, causing them to clump together and reducing their ability to store calcium. This turns the bones brittle and osteoporosis develops. In the joints, the cartilage will degenerate, turn rough and wear away, leading to osteoarthritis. In the thyroid gland, the immune system reacts against degenerating structures. This is how Hashimoto's thyroiditis and Basedow's thyroiditis develop. In the eyes, metabolic waste products are gradually deposited in the lens until cataract forms. The fine structures of the iridocorneal angle degenerate, preventing proper resorption of the aqueous humour and increasing pressure inside the eyes. This leads to development of glaucoma and eventually blindness due to degeneration of the retina (macular degeneration). Storage of proteins that have become insoluble due to oxidative stress (β-amyloids and TAU proteins) in the intercellular substance of the brain, destroys the nerve cells (neurons). Alzheimer's disease develops in such a case. If the regulatory capacity of the biological system collapses, cancer develops because the immune system is no longer able to recognise and eliminate the cancer cells that develop every day.

The immune system recognises all degenerative changes of molecules as foreign so that autoimmune reactions develop, in a failed attempt of the immune system to destroy the seemingly foreign substances, and with the result that the degenerative phenomena are additionally accelerated by autoimmune inflammations, such as the destruction of pancreatic islet cells in type 1 diabetes. This is described in detail in our Bircher-Benner Manual No. 7 for diabetics.

We have seen how excessive (uneconomic) salt intake will damage the endothelium of the blood vessels and the entire condition and structure of the vessels as a result, thereby contributing significantly to the development of hypertension and cardiovascular diseases. This clearly reflects the enormous relevance of the qualitative composition of food: food economy.

The Integral Law of Nutrition[55]

The composition of the ingredients of the plant foods stipulated by Nature corresponds most precisely to the biologically essential requirements. It must be noted that various parts of the plants – the flowers, fruits, kernels, nuts, leaves, stems and roots – contain various substances. The toxic parts must be avoided. If this is taken into account, the requirements of food economy are most readily met if the plant is regarded in its entirety, and if all parts are taken into account in one's everyday diet. The diet should contain fruits, leaves, stems, roots and seeds (taken as whole as possible).

Vibrancy of Food

As we have seen, a high energy potential – a high proportion of fresh food from plants that are capable of photosynthesis – is of great importance in the fight against all degenerative diseases due to its regenerative effect thanks to the high content of biological information from the sunlight stored in the photons. Prevention of all degenerative "diseases of civilisation" requires a high proportion (at least 70 %) of fresh plant-based raw food at the beginning of every meal, and is decisive for healing. In this case, vitamin B12 must be supplemented as long as no dairy products are added, as it does not occur in plants. Fresh plant-based food (raw food) has the highest content of bioactive, pharmacologically active plant substances (phytochemicals) and of all other vitamins that protect us against degeneration, hypertension, arteriosclerosis, infections, thromboses and cancer.

Principles of the Bircher-Benner Diet and Order Therapy

The total food volume should be reduced to the minimum requirement with full quality and gentle preparation. Calculated in calories, the diet should not exceed 2200 Kcal, but should be kept so low that the ideal weight is maintained and an overweight person experiences slow but steady weight reduction. See Bircher-Benner Manual No. 26 healthy and slim, manual for treatment of weight problems, overweight and anorexia. Overeating, even to a small extent, is always harmful because caloric overeating creates insulin and leptin resistance. It must be borne in mind that the calorie calculation is not a qualitative effective food energy, but only a combustion energy. Our diet is adjusted to the energy potential ordering the biological system and vital substances in food economy and content so that it does not contain too much or too little of anything for the cells and the metabolism. As a result, the need for food calculated in calories is considerably lower. See the chapters on food energy and food economy.

The ratio of nutrients should be 45 % slowly degradable carbohydrates, 35 % high-quality vegetable fats (lipids with polyunsaturated fatty acids) and 20 % protein. At the beginning of a treatment of hypertension, the diet should consist of 100 % fresh plant-based food (raw food). Later, a percentage of up to 30 % of cooked whole foods may be allowed. Table salt must be replaced by aromatic spices and fresh herbs to the extent possible. All irritants should be avoided since they cause oxidative stress and increase blood pressure. A daily hike of at least one hour is required. If this is not possible due to pain or disabilities, a different type of movement must be found.

Treatment of hypertension requires an orderly lifestyle, with at least three hours of sleep before midnight. One can easily be active early in the morning. The hormone levels are adjusted to the natural day and the position of the sun.

Mental health issues have an unfavourable effect on diabetes. Relationship conflicts must be cleared up; fears, captivity in a spider's web of relationship conflicts, hatred and feelings of guilt must be healed. A harmonious lifestyle and a light, cheerful mind are highly relevant for healing.

It is very important that people suffering from hypertension understand the diet we teach them is not ours but must become their own. Only then will they succeed in recognising and bearing the necessary responsibility for themselves. We often have an initial tendency to eat beyond what we really need. We must be aware that an excess of food and table salt is particularly harmful for people suffering from hypertension.

Our diet leaves no one hungry. Eating too much is guided by conventional desires for hot spices, table salt and sugar. It is important to remember that these desires will soon disappear completely with this diet and give way to a new, more differentiated sense of taste so that one can look forward to every low-salt meal of fresh food. This indicates that a balanced metabolic balance has been achieved. Overweight diabetics experience a slow, steady weight reduction up to the ideal weight.

Underweight people often have cravings for salt. It is not possible to gain weight on a high calorie fattening diet. They have usually already tried that. However, weight gain up to the individual ideal weight is possible with the help of this diet, which is rich in vital substances and is of high quality in terms of food economy and energy. This high-quality composition of the diet is the prerequisite for successful therapy. It is manifested by a decline in blood pressure.

If hypertension has developed already, medication must not simply be discontinued. In this case, it is important to start the diet and to measure blood pressure every day to gradually reduce the medication with your physician as soon as the blood pressure drops. How quickly this is possible will depend on whether the hardening of the blood vessels is already advanced.

Order of Life and Physical Exercise

Patients with hypertension require a healthy order of life even more than healthy people to create the prerequisite for successful treatment. The sleep and dream phases are biologically specified. Deep, restorative sleep is only possible before midnight. Non-REM (rapid eye movement) sleep phases are unlikely to happen later. There are barely any dreams during these sleep phases. All systems, including heart and circulation, are shut down to rest. After midnight in the REM phase, dreams have the purpose of healing mental trauma and giving our consciousness a certain, precisely dosed insight into the world of the subconscious. Only the eyes and the diaphragm (to breathe) continue moving during the REM phases. This partial paralysis prevents sleepwalking. The deep restoration of the non-REM phases is extremely important for nocturnal regeneration and healing. Therefore the night's rest should begin at 9 pm whenever possible. In return, it is possible to get up very early and be active without becoming exhausted. It is very important to plan for a midday rest, during which the circulation can recover.

It is also very important to walk for at least 30 minutes twice a day for physical exercise, and also to go for an evening walk before bed to stimulate the metabolism. It is still generally unknown that scientific studies have shown that steady walking is more effective than strenuous competitive sport in building up one's stamina. A longer hike should be undertaken regularly at the weekend.

Ten minutes of body exercises in the morning and evening with conscious deep breathing are also important.

Swimming or cycling 10 minutes a day should be added in summer, if possible. One should not spend the entire week sitting down and then go on weekend mountain hikes or strenuous cycling tours, competitions or similar, or force a series of singles tennis matches or 18-hole rounds of golf once a week. Daily stamina training best supports the cardiovascular system, muscles, ligaments and tendons, and is most suitable to order the blood circulation and energy balance. On the other hand, sedentary weeks and forced weekend activities mean stress instead of exercise. Physical exercise contributes to mental relaxation and well-being.

This book is a very important addition to Bircher-Benner Manual No. 19 for patients with hypertension, cardiovascular disease and arteriosclerosis, which we recommend reading.

Menus for the Low-Salt Diet, for Patients with Hypertension and Heart Problems

Week Plan for Strict Salt-free, Natrium-low Diet

1st day
Breakfast:
Almond milk muesli
Salt-free wholemeal bread
(Unsalted) butter
Fruits (selection): oranges, pears, apples, cherries, sour cherries, plums, water melons, tangerines, currants (red or black), bananas, dried figs, grapes
Nuts: almonds, hazel nuts, Brazil nut, walnuts
Tea: herbal tea, honey

Lunch:
Fruits: (as above)
Raw vegetables: cauliflower, romaine lettuce
Cooked dishes: beans, hash browns
Banana cream with pennac milk, small amount of cream and honey, or semolina dumplings

Dinner:
As breakfast, with addition of oat soup

2nd day
Breakfast:
The same every day

Lunch:
Fruits
Raw vegetables: kohlrabi, head lettuce
Cooked dishes: vegetable broth (out of onions, leek, green cabbage, potato peels, sorrel),
cauliflower, parsley potatoes

Dinner:
As breakfast, with addition of cereal porridge with grapes

3rd day
Breakfast: (as above)

Lunch:
Fruits
Raw vegetables: parsnip,
head lettuce
Cooked dishes: peas, cooked in rice ring,
fruit jelly prepared with agar-agar

Dinner:
As above, with addition of thick potato soup

4th day
Breakfast: (as above)

Lunch:
Fruits
Raw vegetables: cauliflower, cress
Cooked dishes: oat groat soup,
sautéed kohlrabi, potato puree

Dinner:
Fruits and nuts
Rice porridge
Plum compote

5th day
Breakfast: (as above)

Lunch:
Fruits
Raw vegetables: chicory/endive, green cabbage
Cooked dishes: cooked romaine lettuce,

oat flake dumplings with soy (instead of eggs)
Backed apples (with grapes or nuts)

Dinner:
Same as breakfast

6th day
Breakfast: (as above)

Lunch:
Fruits
Raw vegetables: parsnip, Brussels sprouts
Cooked dishes: onion soup,
sautéed broccoli, caraway potatoes

Dinner: (as above)

7th day
Breakfast: (as above)

Lunch:
Fruits
Raw vegetables: chicory/endive, romaine lettuce
Cooked dishes: sautéed Brussels sprouts, Japanese rice
Chilled banana soup

Dinner:
As above, with addition of salt-free cheese

Menu for 1 Week of Salt-free Diet (Milder Form)

1st day
Fruits, dried fruits
Raw vegetables: carrots, endive/chicory, head lettuce
Vegetable broth with bread cubes without salt
Black salsify with lemon and cream; potatoes with tomatoes

2nd day
Fruits, dried fruits
Raw vegetables: beetroot (red beet), cucumber, cress
Tomatoes, stuffed with rice
Lemon cream

3rd day
Fruits
Raw vegetables: celery root (celeriac), tomatoes, lamb's lettuce
Semolina soup
Chopped cabbage, caraway potatoes

4th day
Fruits
Raw vegetables: black salsify, spinach, endive/chicory
Polenta slices
Apple cream

5th day
Fruits
Raw vegetables: radish, courgettes, head lettuce
Vegetable soup
Swiss chard in sauce, Lyonnaise potatoes

6th day
Fruits
Raw vegetables: cauliflower, cress, head lettuce
Chervil soup
Spinach pasta with tomato sauce and salt-free cheese

7th day
Fruits
Raw vegetables: raw tomatoes stuffed with celery (celeriac) salad and head lettuce
Cooked Jerusalem artichoke with a small amount of lemon juice, potato puree with tomatoes
Semolina pudding with raspberry syrup

Breakfast:
Bircher muesli or fruits or fruit juice
Salt-free bread
Butter or health food store vegetable margarine
Rosehip tea or herbal tea
Nuts, grated or whole

Dinner:
Fruits or fruit salad or grapefruit
or Bircher muesli
with soup, bread and salt-free cheese
or baked potatoes with herb quark and salad
or sandwiches and salad etc.

Recipes for Salt-free and Low-salt Food

These are very important for the prevention and cure of salt-sensitive hypertension as well as for kidney disease and hypertension of the eye (glaucoma). If signs of arteriosclerosis are already present (e.g. in the form of angina pectoris or documented constrictions in any other arteries), recipes with eggs should be avoided and health food fat or olive oil should be used instead of butter. Bircher-Benner Manual No. 19 for patients with hypertension, cardiovascular disease and arteriosclerosis provides detailed information on this.

If pre-existing hypertension needs to be cured, a strict raw food diet should be followed for several weeks to months, as explained and described in detail in our Manual No. 4 for fresh juices, raw vegetables and fruit dishes.

Juices

Juices are "raw fruits and vegetables" in a mechanically refined form as an additional special enrichment and when coarse food (cellulose) is not permitted. Whole raw vegetables are always of a higher nutritional quality and thus cannot be permanently replaced by juice.

For the preparation of juices, raw fruits and vegetables must be cleaned thoroughly, pressed with a hand press or an electric centrifugal juicer, and served immediately. Letting them stand reduces their value.

If a small hand press is used, fruits and vegetables must be chopped first. Finely grate apples, pears and all bulb vegetables, and finely chop leafy vegetables and herbs.

Fruit juices
Single fruit juices:
Orange, tangerine, grapefruit, apple, pear, grape, strawberry, blueberry, currant, blackcurrant, raspberry, peach, apricot, plum, mango, Japanese persimmon (kaki), kiwi
Mixed fruit juices:
Citrus fruit only to be used if there is no hypersensitivity to them.
For example, orange, tangerine, grapefruit, Japanese persimmon (kaki) or berry juice mixed with apple juice; or berry juice mixed with peach, apricot or plum juice; or whipped bananas mixed with orange, berry, peach, mango or apricot juice

Additions to taste or as needed: lemon juice, honey, maple syrup, fruit concentrate, cream, yoghurt, almond milk, flaxseed, rice or barley gruel

Vegetable juices
When fresh they have a high mineral and vitamin content. Each juice has its own special nutritional value.

Single vegetable juices
Tomato, carrot, beetroot (red beet), radish, cabbage, celery root (celeriac), all leafy vegetables, bulb and root vegetables juice; stinging nettle, sorrel and dandelion juice for springtime blood-cleansing treatment

Mixed vegetable juices
Carrot, tomato, and spinach in equal proportions (very good flavour)

Tomatoes and carrots
Tomatoes and spinach

Other mixes (and cocktails) can be combined according to taste.

For variety add sorrel, stinging nettle, chives, parsley, onions, tender celery (celeriac) leaves or roots, and other herbs.

Additions per glass (1 ½–2 dl): 1 tbs cream, almond puree or buttermilk, a touch of lemon juice, fruit concentrate (optional, small quantity). Flaxseed (optional), rice or barley gruel. Other leafy vegetables or lettuces may also be used, such as white cabbage, endive/chicory, lamb's lettuce, romaine lettuce or dandelion.

Potato juice
Prepare well-cleaned, peeled (optional) potatoes (must not be unripe, green or germinated) in the same manner as carrots for carrot juice. Potato juice is unpleasant to drink, and should be consumed in small quantities and only when prescribed by a doctor. Adding apple juice (one apple) improves the taste.

Gruel Added to Juices

The gruel is added to raw juices at ⅓; it neutralises the sharpness of the fruit or vegetable flavour. The gruel for one day can be prepared once a day and kept in the thermos flask until use.

a) Rice or barley gruel:
   Stir 1 heaped tsp of rice or barley wholemeal flour with 2 dl cold water and boil stirring constantly for 5 minutes. Let cool.

b) Flaxseed gruel:
   Wash 1 tbs flaxseeds, boil in 2 dl water for 10 minutes, strain and let cool.

Bircher Muesli

All recipes are for 1 person.

Apple muesli
The original apple muesli, as first introduced by Dr Bircher, is still the best food diet and has been used thousandfold on his own patients. This tried-and-tested food diet is based on our many years' experience.

In general the best apples are both sweet and tart, white-fleshed and juicy, e.g. Klar, Gravenstein, Sauergrauech, Menznauer Jäger, Jonathan, Ontario, Rubinette, Glockenäpfel, Braeburn, Topaz, Champagner-Reinetten, Cox's Orange and Granny Smith.

If apples are dry or tasteless, their aroma can be enriched by adding a small amount of freshly grated zest of untreated organic oranges or lemons, or orange juice or rose hip puree, or of freshly grated ginger.

Apple muesli with yoghurt, sour milk or buttermilk
1 tbs oat flakes
3 tbs water
2 tbs Bifidus yoghurt or
Bifidus sour milk or buttermilk
1 tsp honey
200 g apples
1 tbs hazelnuts or almonds, ground

Soak the oat flakes for 12 hours (overnight for breakfast). Mix the oat flakes, yoghurt (or sour milk) and honey until smooth. Remove the stems and calyxes from the washed apples, and using the Bircher grater grate the apples into the mixture. Stir several times to keep the muesli attractively white. Spread nuts on top and always serve at once.

Versions: Replace oat flakes with wheat, rice, barley, rye, semolina, buckwheat or soy flakes, optionally mixed with yeast flakes (to enrich the muesli with vitamin B).

Another version: Mix 1 tsp soaked oat flakes with 1 tsp cereal grains (whole, coarse-ground or mixed; soak in water for 24 hours then pass through a sieve and rinse with cold water). Instead of being grated, the apples can be worked in with a hand blender.

Apple muesli with almond or sesame puree *(vegan)*
For use when animal protein is prohibited in the case of allergies.
1 tbs oat flakes
3 tbs water
½ tbs lemon juice
1 tbs almond or sesame puree
1 tbs honey
3 tbs water
200 g apples
1 tbs hazelnuts or almonds, ground

Soak oat flakes for 12 hours. Stir in lemon juice, puree, honey and water, and whisk to a creamy consistency. Add the oat flakes and apples (prepared like basic recipe). Spread nuts on top and serve immediately.

Apple muesli with cream
Specially enriched recipe designed for weight gain. For diabetics, without honey and without oat flakes.
1 tbs (8 g) fine oat flakes
3 tbs water
½ tbs lemon juice
3–4 tbs cream
1 tbs honey
200 g apples
1 tbs hazelnuts or almonds, ground

Prepared as for basic recipe.

Muesli with berries and stone fruit
Particularly rich in vitamin C.
Prepare an almond puree, sesame puree or yoghurt dressing.
At the end add:
150–200 g strawberries or raspberries, blueberries, currants or blackberries, mash coarsely with a fork
or
150–200 g plums, peaches or apricots, pitted and passed through a blender or cut finely with a knife.

Muesli with various fruits
The following combinations are very tasty:
Strawberries and raspberries
Strawberries, raspberries and currants
Strawberries and apples
Blackberries and apples
Apples with finely cut orange and tangerine segments
Apples and bananas
Apples and peaches
Dressing with almond or sesame puree, or yoghurt.
Use only fresh fruits, never tinned (fruit salad, etc.).

Muesli with dried fruits
If you have no fresh fruits at hand, you can make the muesli using dried fruits (apples, apricots, plums, pears). Wash and soak 100 g of dried fruits in cold water for 12 hours, and pass through the blender. Mix with almond or sesame puree or yoghurt dressing. For dried fruits, always look for high quality without preservatives or bleach; otherwise gastrointestinal problems may occur.

Muesli with condensed milk
If you do not have almond or sesame puree or fresh yoghurt at hand, you can make the muesli with condensed milk according to the original recipe. Disadvantage: condensed milk often contains sugar. Condensed milk was used in the original recipe because bovine tuberculo-

sis was prevalent at the time. That is why babies were also fed condensed milk.

Raw Vegetables and Salads

The following three basic rules should be observed when preparing raw vegetables and salads:

1. Freshness and quality
For the diet without or with only a small amount of table salt (as for all diets and for a normal everyday nutrition), use only sun-ripened, organically grown vegetables and salads. They are not only ideal for health, but also taste best. Today the supply from producers who work in accordance with organic guidelines is very extensive, and organic vegetables are available in many supermarkets. Vegetables and salads from your own garden are ideal, of course. Herbs and tomatoes can be grown even on a balcony. Choose young, tender leafy lettuces and root vegetables, unblanched, and remove any wilted leaves or rotting stalks. For a healing regime, it is important to use only the freshest plants of the highest quality.
Prepare raw vegetables just before mealtime, then mix them immediately with the dressing. Unless eaten immediately, chopped vegetables and salads lose much of their vitamin content.

2. Thorough cleaning
Organic vegetables without manure fertilisation contain no worm eggs. Nevertheless, all fresh plants must be cleaned thoroughly and carefully. Note that water-soluble substances such as vitamin C, B-group vitamins and minerals are leached out in water.

3. Harmonious composition
Every salad dish should contain all three types of vegetables: root, fruit and leaf. Green leafy lettuce in particular is always part of a healing regime. Concerning the dressings, variety is desirable for the various ingredients of the raw food diet.
A beautifully assembled salad in pleasing colours is agreeable to the eye and the palate, and it stimulates the appetite. Small garnishes of herbs, radishes, young carrots or olives make the raw vegetable dish even more colourful and festive. In everyday life, serve no more than the three kinds of vegetables per meal. Too much variety may impair digestion.

Cleaning leafy vegetables
For head lettuce, endive/chicory, romaine lettuce, iceberg lettuce and similar green leaf lettuces, cabbage and red cabbage, etc.: Separate the leaves and clean them individually and carefully under running water. Rinse several times and dry thoroughly in a salad spinner.
Small-leaved salads such as lamb's lettuce and cut lettuce, spinach, dandelion, cress, rocket, radicchio and Brussel sprouts should be rinsed repeatedly in small portions, with any root or hard stalks removed.
Halve endive/chicory and radicchio, remove outer leaves and rinse thoroughly.

Cleaning root vegetables
Celery root (celeriac), carrots, horseradish, radishes, beetroot (red beet), kohlrabi and salsify. Clean with a brush under running water, peel and immediately grate or slice into the finished dressing. Mix well to preserve the vegetables' fresh colour.

Cleaning vegetable fruits
Wash tomatoes and cut them into wedges or slices. Peel cucumbers and cut them small or grate them. Organic young cucumbers do not need to be peeled.
Use only young, tender unpeeled courgettes for salads, wash them thoroughly then slice or julienne.
Green and yellow sweet peppers are milder than the red variety. Wash, halve, remove seeds and dice. Only use organic

sweet peppers, as unfortunately almost all non-organic sweet peppers now come from hydroponic production.
Separate cauliflower and broccoli into florets and clean thoroughly under running water.
Wash celery stalks, peel, and cut away hard parts.
Halve leeks and fennel and rinse under the spray tap.

Salad Dressings

The quantities are calculated for 1 person. All dressings for salads and raw vegetables are prepared without salt. We can replace salt with fresh kitchen herbs, onions, soy products (e.g. Miro), Kelpamare or pressed garlic (optional).

Preparation of raw vegetables
It is important to always prepare the salad and raw vegetable dressings first, then grate, slice or cut the carefully washed leaves or roots directly into the dressing and toss the salad immediately. This limits value loss from exposure to atmospheric oxygen to the unavoidable minimum. This is particularly evident in grated apples and celery root (celeriac), which quickly change colour without dressing but remain beautifully white when mixed with dressing. Salads and raw vegetables should not be left standing for long; they should be eaten as quickly as possible.

Oil dressing
1 tbs oil (rapeseed, sunflower or olive oil from first cold pressing, thistle oil, walnut oil)
Always add $1/3$ flaxseed oil.
1 tsp lemon juice or organic fruit vinegar
Small clove of garlic, pressed (optional)
1 tsp fresh herbs (or pinch of dried herbs)

Mix all the ingredients and whisk the dressing until creamy. The dressing is even tastier with a splash of soy sauce or Kelpamare.
This classic salad dressing is suitable for all green salads (head lettuce, romaine lettuce, cress, etc.) and fruit salads (tomatoes, cucumbers, etc.)

Quark-yoghurt dressing
For low-fat diet.

1 tbs low-fat quark
3 tbs yoghurt or sour milk
½ tsp lemon juice
Fresh, finely chopped herbs
Finely chopped onion or pressed garlic

Whisk all ingredients thoroughly.
This dressing goes particularly well with root vegetables, e.g. carrots, celery root (celeriac), radish.

Yoghurt dressing
For low-fat diet.

2–3 tbs yoghurt
A few drops of lemon juice
Onion, grated (optional)
Small clove of garlic, pressed (optional)
1 tsp fresh herbs (or pinch of dried herbs)

Whisk all ingredients thoroughly.
A refreshing dressing with cress or spinach, with fruit salads (tomatoes, cucumbers) and with root vegetables (kohlrabi, radish, radishes).

Cream dressing
2 tbs sour cream
1 tsp low-fat quark
1 tsp lemon juice
Small amount of pepper
1 tsp fresh herbs (or pinch of dried herbs)

Whisk all ingredients thoroughly. This dressing goes well with almost all root and fruit salads. For variety you may replace lemon juice with orange juice to give the raw food a new flavour. For celery root (celeriac), beetroot (red beet) and endive/chicory salad you may add a small amount of freshly ground horseradish to the dressing for a very stimulating taste.

Almond puree or sesame puree dressing
(vegan)
Diet without animal protein.

1 tbs almond or sesame puree
3 tbs water
1 tsp lemon juice
Small clove of garlic, pressed (optional)
1 tsp fresh herbs (or pinch of dried herbs)

Slowly stir sesame or almond puree with water until smooth, then add the other ingredients.
This tasty dressing is perfect for root vegetables.

Mayonnaise, classic recipe
For 4 persons:

1 egg yolk
1 tbs lemon juice
2 dl oil
Onion, herbs and a small amount of Kelpamare

Mix the egg yolk well with several drops of lemon juice. Add the oil drop by drop while whisking evenly. If the mayonnaise becomes too thick, dilute with lemon juice. Season to taste, without table salt.

For 1 portion:
1 tbs mayonnaise
1 tsp lemon juice
1 tsp fresh herbs (or pinch of dried herbs)
Mix all ingredients thoroughly.

Mayonnaise with wholemeal soy flour instead of egg
Recipe for vegan nutrition or the exclusion of animal protein.
For 6–8 persons:

2 tbs soy wholemeal flour
6 tbs water
2 dl oil

Mix soy wholemeal flour and water until smooth. Slowly add oil while constantly stirring with the whisk.
The mayonnaise can be kept in the refrigerator for several days.

For 1 portion:
1 tbs mayonnaise
1 tsp lemon juice
Dab of mustard (optional)
1 tsp fresh herbs (or pinch of dried herbs)

Mix all ingredients well.

Mayonnaise is a popular dressing for salads composed of fruit vegetables and root vegetables.

Quark mayonnaise
1 tbs cream or low-fat quark
1–2 tbs milk
If desired: 1 yolk
1–2 tbs oil
½ tsp diet mustard
1 tsp lemon juice
Small amount of Kelpamare
Fresh chopped herbs

Stir quark and milk until smooth, add egg yolk to refine (optional). Add oil, mustard and lemon juice and whisk well. Season with Kelpamare and herbs.

Spicy quark dressing
For persons not sensitive to fat.

1 tbs quark
3 tbs yoghurt or 1 tbs cream and 2 tbs yoghurt

1 tsp soy meal or
1 egg yolk
1 tbs lemon juice
Small amount of horseradish
or nutmeg and curry
½ apple, finely grated
Cress or chervil, chopped
½ tsp fruit concentrate or
buckhorn pulp

Stir and mix all ingredients well, vary seasoning according to taste.

Sweet and sour salad dressings
For variety each salad dressing can be seasoned sweet and sour by adding fruit juice concentrate, pear syrup (Birnel), honey or tomato paste. Sour milk, mixed with fruit juice concentrate or Birnel, also makes a low-fat dressing that is well suited for carrot or leaf salads.

Raw vegetables, mixed
Chicory/endive with diced tomato – oil dressing or mayonnaise
Sweet pepper and fennel – oil dressing
Fennel, chicory/endive and diced tomato – mayonnaise
Fennel and carrots – cream dressing
Cauliflower and carrots – cream dressing
Tomatoes and sweet pepper – oil dressing or mayonnaise

These mixed salads must be chewed thoroughly. In case of nausea, serve without dressing.

Tomatoes raw, stuffed
With cucumbers – oil dressing or mayonnaise
With celery root (celeriac) – cream dressing
With cauliflower – cream dressing

Celery root (celeriac)-apple-banana raw food
20 g quark
3 tbs cream or yoghurt
Juice of ½ lemon
200 g finely diced apples
100 g banana slices
50 g grated celery root (celeriac)
Small amount of walnuts

Stir quark with cream or yoghurt, add the other ingredients and mix well. Add yoghurt if the mix becomes too dry. Garnish with walnuts.

Sprouted cereal grains
These have a very high amount of vitamins in groups E and B, and generally provide a strengthening effect.

Wheat, rye, oats, barley.
1st day, dinner: Wash the grains in a colander under running water and place them in a bowl. Cover with water. Keep at room temperature, close to the oven.
2nd day, breakfast: Rinse the grains and spread to dry on a flat plate. Keep at room temperature, close to the oven.
Dinner: Put the grains back in the bowl and cover with water. Keep at room temperature, close to the oven.
3rd day, breakfast: Rinse the grains and spread to dry on the plate.
Dinner: Put the grains back in the bowl and cover with water. Keep at room temperature, close to the oven.
The grains should have developed sprouts 1–2 cm long.

As baby food
Shredded soaked cereal mixed with bananas, honey and water.

Sauerkraut salad
Sauerkraut is a particularly wholesome raw vegetable, especially in winter. It is more easily digestible raw than cooked and has a gallbladder-purging and disinfecting effect. It is imperative to use low-salt organic sauerkraut. An addition of finely cut raw sauerkraut can considerably improve the taste and digestive qualities of steamed sauerkraut. For a salad, the sauerkraut is loosely separated and

chopped, mixed with a few caraway seeds (or ground caraway), 3–4 chopped juniper berries, chopped onion, and a julienned apple or small fresh diced pineapple. Choose oil dressing as a garnish. This salad goes particularly well with lamb's lettuce (corn salad) and a raw root vegetable.

Mixed and pureed raw vegetables
If the doctor prescribes a "pureed diet", certain raw vegetables may be mixed with the dressing in the blender. This is the transition from juice to normal raw vegetable food.

Examples:
1 tomato 70 g, 1 handful spinach 30 g, 1 small carrot 70 g, pinch of marjoram, oil dressing

1 tomato 70 g, 1 handful head lettuce 20 g, 1 small piece of celery root (celeriac) 20 g, cream dressing (season with lovage)

Beetroot (red beet) 30 g, courgette 40 g, head lettuce 20 g, cream dressing (with dill)

Celery root (celeriac) 40 g, carrots 40 g, spinach 20 g, almond puree dressing (season with rosemary)

Vegetables that can be eaten raw and the matching herbs and dressings

Spices
Fresh wild and culinary herbs are rich in vital substances and, when well dosed, provide a rich variety of taste and aroma in food and raw salads. They stimulate the appetite and digestive secretion.

Chopped onions, garlic, grated horseradish, ginger, cardamom, Kelpamare and soy spices (e.g. miso) from the health food store also enrich dishes with their valuable content and aroma.

Pungent spices such as mustard, chili, pepper and curry should only be used in small amounts, since too strong a stimulation of the digestive juices may cause thirst, nausea, stomach burning, indigestion and headaches.

Suggestions for Dressings to go with Salads and Raw Vegetables

Head lettuce	uncut	oil dressing	chives, onion
Leaf lettuce	uncut	oil dressing	chives, onion
Endive/chicory	cut in strips of 1 cm	oil dressing	onion, parsley
Lamb's lettuce	uncut	oil dressing	onion, parsley
Cress	uncut	yoghurt dressing	chives
Spinach	cut in strips of ½ cm	yoghurt dressing	peppermint
Cabbage salads: white cabbage, sauerkraut, Brussel sprouts, savoy cabbage	slice, cut into thin pieces	oil dressing or nut dressing	lovage, thyme, savory, caraway
Tomatoes	slice or dice	oil dressing or yoghurt dressing	basil, thyme, oregano
Cucumber	slice	oil dressing	dill
Fennel	cut thin with knife	cream dressing or oil dressing	dill, chives, parsley

Sweet pepper	cut into fine strips	oil dressing or mayonnaise	chives
Radish	slice or grate	quark dressing	chives, parsley
Radishes	slice or cut finely	yoghurt dressing	chives, parsley
Celery stalks	cut finely	oil dressing or almond puree dressing	chives, thyme
Courgette	grate coarsely or slice	oil dressing or almond puree dressing	dill, borage, basil
Carrots	grate finely	yoghurt or orange dressing	chives, lovage
Celery root (celeriac)	grate finely	nut dressing	ginger
Beetroot (red beet)	grate finely	cream dressing	horseradish
Cauliflower, broccoli	cut off florets, grate stems	garlic dressing	chives
Chicory/endive	cut in strips of 1 cm	cream dressing	tarragon, parsley
Jerusalem artichoke	grate	mayonnaise	marjoram, thyme
Kohlrabi	slice or grate	yoghurt dressing or nut dressing	thyme, lovage
Red cabbage	slice or cut finely	almond puree dressing	grated apple, caraway, lovage

Chives, parsley and onions may be added in moderation to any raw vegetable, according to taste.

Milk Types

Almond milk
Vegetable nutrition with protein and oil, rich in unsaturated vegetable oils. It calms the lining of the stomach and intestines through its milky mildness.
1 tbs almond puree
1 tsp honey
1½ water and ½ dl fruit juice (thickens slightly)

Whisk almond puree and honey and add the water drop by drop. Add the fruit juice last.

Almond milk from fresh almonds
Very easy to digest.

1½ tbs almonds, peeled (no bitter ones)
1 tsp honey
1½ dl water

Mix almonds, honey and water in the mixer, strain, if necessary.

Pine nut milk
Very rich in easily digestible, metabolically gentle vegetable oils and proteins.

1 tbs pine nuts, washed
1 tsp honey
1½ dl water

Prepare like almond milk.

Sesame milk
2 dl water (cold or warm)
1 level tbs sesame paste
1 tsp lemon juice
1 tsp honey

Whisk sesame paste and honey and add the water drop by drop, adding the lemon juice last.

Sesame cream
Like sesame milk, with less added water. For cooked food and desserts as a cream substitute.

Sesame frappé (shake)
Like sesame milk or sesame cream, with addition of fruit juice, apple juice, fruit concentrates.

Soy milk
1 cup soy beans
7 cups water
1 tbs fruit sugar
Water

Wash and dry soy beans and grind them in an almond mill. Soak for 2 hours then boil for 20 minutes in the same water used for soaking, stirring constantly. Strain. Add water until the viscosity of cow's milk is reached. Add fruit sugar, leave to cool.
Soy milk is available in tetra packs in health food stores.

Butter, Vegetable Fats and Oils

The Bircher kitchen uses only cold-pressed oils, almond puree and other nut spreads for raw food. Cooked food may also be prepared using small amounts of fresh butter, olive oil and unhardened vegetable fats from health food stores. Vegetable oils generally should not be heated, since the unsaturated fatty acids may turn into dangerous radicals. Only olive oil may be heated to 170 °C, as it contains monounsaturated fatty acids.

Fresh butter
To refine the dishes.

Health food store vegetable margarine and food fats
Such products in Switzerland include Nussella, Becel, Olima; in Germany they include Vitaquell and Eden.

These are vegetable fat emulsions from naturally solid (i.e. unhardened) fats such as coconut oil or palm kernel oil, in combination with the highest possible proportion of liquid oils and seed oils, particularly sunflower or olive oil. The ratio of omega-3 fatty acids to omega-6 fatty acids must be at least 1:5. Since sunflower oil contains almost no omega-3 fatty acids, one-third flaxseed oil must be added at all times. This also applies to olive oil. Omega-6 fatty acids stimulate the Th-II pathway of CD-4 helper cells and therefore promote inflammatory responses. Omega-3 fatty acids, on the other hand, modulate the immune system and are particularly important in the defence against cancer.

More on this subject can be found in the Bircher-Benner Manual No. 4 for fresh juices, raw vegetables and fruit dishes.

Nut spread and almond puree
These have a delicate, nutty flavour. They can be used diversely in a light diet or to replace fresh butter or vegetable margarine served with vegetables, potatoes, rice and pasta products.

Sunflower oil (cold-pressed), maize-germ oil, safflower oil, flaxseed oil, olive oil (cold-pressed)
Organic and rich in unsaturated fatty acids, these oils are more easily digestible for most people than heated butter. However, as mentioned, vegetable oils should not be heated since they may then release dangerous radicals that promote oxidative stress and thus degenerative processes and the development of cancer cells. Flaxseed takes slightly bitter. However, it mixes well with Bircher muesli and salad

dressings. If the taste is too strong, the oil is rancid and should no longer be used. Adding a small amount of lemon juice it is suitable for certain raw vegetables, such as carrots and celery root (celeriac). Particularly recommended as anti-oxidative cure with 2–4 tbs per day. Do not leave the oil container open, but keep it tightly closed in the fridge. Adding lemon juice protects against oxidation.

Gentle Cooking and Steaming

Few housewives or working woman today will want to do without their pressure cookers. This is time-saving and even healthier, since it is not heated up for as long and fewer nutrients are extracted with the cooking water. Who wouldn't want these advantages?

The pressure cooker is very helpful especially for soups for almost every recipe. The cooking time in the pressure cooker is only $1/3$–$1/4$ of the usual time.

Many vegetable and potato recipes can be steamed gently in the pressure cooker. This will result in dishes that retain their colour, flavour, vitamins and nutrients, and that cook much faster. The cooking time of vegetables (except potatoes) can be reduced even with conventional steaming if you like your vegetables a little crunchier, i.e. al dente.

For cereal dishes, it is recommended to use the steamer for foods with long cooking times (e.g. wholegrain rice, millet, barley, coarse corn), but not for pasta products.

Soups

All recipes are for 1 person:

The following soup and vegetable recipes require a large amount of vegetable broth. In a small household, it is inconvenient to make fresh vegetable broth every day. Instead, you may use ordinary water and vegetable stock (available salt-free) in cubes or pastes. Ensure that there is no glutamate or yeast extract contained. Many people are allergic to yeast and other fungi, including baker's yeast. Cream improves all soups and vegetables, but milk can be used in most cases.

In case of wheat allergy, the wholemeal flour in the recipes can be replaced by rice, millet or oat flour. Intolerance to milk protein is very common today because of the industrial processing of milk (i.e. homogenisation).

Vegetable broth
This recipe is for 4 persons:

1 tbs health food store vegetable fat
1 onion
2 carrots
1 small celery root (celeriac) (150 g)*
Cabbage, Swiss chard leaves
1 leek stalk
3–4 l water
½ bay leaf
Lovage, basil or
other herbs, preferably fresh, otherwise dried.

Halve the onion, keeping the brown peel, and brown the cut area in the hot fat or olive oil. Chop the vegetables, add and cook covered for at least 15 minutes at low heat. Add water and cook for 2 hours at low heat. Season to taste but use a minimum of salt*.

* Table salt must be avoided altogether on a strictly sodium-free diet. Vegetable broth tastes good even then.

Vegetable stock
3 dl vegetable broth
Small amount of Kelpamare (optional)
10 g nut spread or health food store vegetable fat
Parsley, chives, freshly chopped herbs

Prepare the vegetable broth according to the above recipe and add to nut spread or vegetable fat and herbs. Season with Kelpamare (optional).

Soup Additions

Butter dumplings
½ tbs butter
1 tbs flour
¼ dl milk, hot
½ egg
Lovage, basil, marjoram, parsley, chives, marjoram, nutmeg (optional)

Sauté the flour in the butter, add hot milk and beat until the mixture separates from the pan. Whisk the egg and beat it into the hot batter.
With a teaspoon place the dumplings in the boiling stock and allow to simmer gently for 5 minutes. Season but do not salt.

Pancake strips
1 tbs flour
½ egg
½ dl milk
½ dl water
1 tbs health food store vegetable fat
Sage (finely chopped) or sorrel leaves or mint leaves, chives, parsley, a small amount of nutmeg (optional)

Prepare a thin batter from flour, egg, milk and water; season. Cook a pancake in vegetable fat and cut it into fine strips.

Semolina dumplings
10 g butter
1 ½ tbs fine semolina
½–1 egg
Marjoram, nutmeg

Whip the butter until frothy. Mix the semolina and egg thoroughly with the butter and leave to stand for 30 minutes. Use a tsp to shape the dumplings. Place them in the boiling vegetable stock and steep for 15–20 minutes.

Rice soup, clear
½ tbs health food store vegetable fat
Small amount of chopped onion
1 small carrot
Small amount of celery root (celeriac)*
and leek
1 tbs rice
6 dl vegetable broth
Chives

Sauté onion with finely cut vegetables and rice. Add hot vegetable broth and cook for 15–20 minutes. Prepare with finely cut chives and vegetable fat.

* Omit if on a strictly sodium-free diet.

Rice soup, thickened
½ tbs health food store vegetable fat
Small amount of celery root (celeriac)*
1 small carrot
Small amount of leek
1 tbs rice
½ tbs wholemeal flour
6 dl vegetable broth or water
Lovage, parsley, basil, marjoram
Dash of soya sauce (optional)
½ tbs cream or sesame cream (see recipe page 38)
Chives

Sauté the diced vegetables and rice in the vegetable fat. Sprinkle with wholemeal flour, add the vegetable broth and cook for 30 minutes. Season with soy sauce and herbs. Place cream and finely cut chives in soup bowl and pour the soup over them.

Herbal soup
1 tbs wholemeal flour
1 dl milk or water
5 dl vegetable broth
½ tbs cream
5 g butter or vegetable margarine or nut spread or
1 egg yolk (optional)

Lovage, basil, marjoram, parsley, chives, nutmeg or caraway (optional)

Stir wholemeal flour into cold milk or cold water and add to the boiling vegetable broth. Cook for 15 minutes. Season with the herbs. Put cream or (optional) butter, vegetable margarine, nut spread or egg yolk into the soup bowl, add the soup and whisk.

Oat cream soup
½ tbs health food store vegetable fat
2 tbs fine or coarse oat flakes
6 dl vegetable broth
Small amount of celery root (celeriac)*
½ tbs cream or sesame cream (see recipe page 38)
Small amount of miso (optional)
Chives, nutmeg or caraway (optional)

Briefly sauté oat flakes with or without vegetable fat. Add vegetable broth and celery root (celeriac). Simmer fine oat flakes for 10 minutes or coarse oat flakes for at least 20 minutes. Season to taste. Place cream or sesame cream and chives in the soup bowl and add the pureed soup.

* Omit if on a strictly sodium-free diet.

Oat groat soup
½ tbs health food store vegetable fat
2 tbs oat groats
Small amount of chopped onion
7 dl water or vegetable broth
1 dl milk
Small amount of celery root (celeriac)*, finely diced
Small amount of miso
1 tbs cream (optional)
Chives, parsley, marjoram or borage

Sauté onion and groats with or without vegetable fat. Add vegetable broth, milk and celery root (celeriac) and cook for 45–60 minutes. Season to taste with a small amount of miso. Place cream

and herbs in the soup bowl and add the soup.

* Omit if on a strictly sodium-free diet.

Semolina soup
1 tbs semolina
5 dl vegetable broth
½ tbs cream or sesame cream (see recipe page 38)
1 egg yolk or
5 g fresh butter or vegetable fat or nut spread
Small amount of Kelpamare (optional)
Caraway, nutmeg (optional)
Lovage, basil, marjoram, parsley, chives

Stir semolina into the boiling vegetable broth, add Kelpamare and caraway, and simmer for 30 minutes. Season to taste with herbs. Place cream and egg yolk (alternatively butter, vegetable fat or nut spread) in the soup bowl and add the soup.

Tomato soup
½ tbs health food store vegetable fat
Small amount of onion and leek
1 small carrot
1 garlic clove
1 tomato
1 tbs wholemeal flour
6 dl vegetable broth
Small amount of tomato puree (optional)
Pinch of fruit sugar (or Succanat)
Rosemary, oregano
5 g butter, vegetable margarine or nut spread
½ tbs cream or sesame cream (see recipe page 38)
Chives

Sauté vegetables (cut small) with or without vegetable fat, then add the tomato. Sprinkle with wholemeal flour and pour the vegetable broth into the mixture. Simmer for 30 minutes then strain. Add spices and tomato puree (optional). Place butter or vegetable fat (or nut spread) and cream in the soup bowl and add the finished soup. Sprinkle with finely cut chives. If desired, add 1 tbs wholegrain rice to the soup or sprinkle with croutons toasted without vegetable fat.

Summer tomato soup
4 ripe summer tomatoes
Pinch of fruit sugar (or Succanat)
1 tbs sea salt*
1 tbs cream

Dice the tomatoes, cook briefly, season and strain. Add cream and serve the soup lukewarm or cold.

* Omit if on a salt-free diet.

Vegetable soups (carrots, spinach, broccoli, cauliflower)
½ tbs health food store vegetable fat
Small amount of chopped onion
1 ½ tbs wholemeal flour
5 dl vegetable broth
1 dl milk
1 tbs cream or sesame cream (see recipe page 38)

Vegetables: 1 diced carrot or 1 small cup of spinach, pureed or finely chopped, broccoli or cauliflower finely chopped (cook some of the flowers separately and set them aside).

Sauté onion and carrots or broccoli or cauliflower with or without vegetable fat. Sprinkle with wholemeal flour and sauté briefly. Pour in vegetable broth and milk, and simmer for 20–40 minutes. For the spinach soup, add the spinach last and remove from heat. Pour the soup over the cream in the soup bowl. For the broccoli and cauliflower soup, add the florets previously set aside.
Seasoning the vegetable soups:
For carrot soup, use lovage, rosemary or marjoram, and 1 tsp caraway.

For spinach soup, use a small amount of peppermint leaves, parsley, chives and a pinch of nutmeg.
For broccoli or cauliflower soup, use a small amount of basil, parsley, chives and tarragon.

Chervil soup
½ tbs health food store vegetable fat
Small amount of onion
1 medium-sized potato, diced
½ tbs wholemeal flour
5 dl vegetable broth
1 tbs chervil, chopped
1 tbs cream

Sauté the onion slightly with or without vegetable fat. Add potato, sprinkle with wholemeal flour and add vegetable broth. Cook for 30 minutes and strain. Put chervil and cream in the soup bowl and add the soup.

Leek cream soup
½ tbs health food store vegetable fat
¼ leek
1 ½ tbs flour
6 dl vegetable broth
1 tbs cream
1 yolk (optional)
Nutmeg

Sauté the roughly chopped leeks in the vegetable fat until they soften. Sprinkle the flour on top, add the vegetable broth and cook for 30–45 minutes. Strain, season with nutmeg. Add 1 tbs of cream and 1 egg yolk (optional) to the soup bowl and pour the soup over it.

Onion soup
½ tbs health food store vegetable fat
1 onion
1 tbs flour
5 dl water or vegetable broth
1 tsp nut spread
Small amount of Kelpamare
Basil, nutmeg

Cut the onions into fine strips and sauté in the vegetable margarine until soft. Sprinkle flour over the onion and sauté briefly. Add water or vegetable broth and cook for 30 minutes. Season to taste. Place nut spread in the soup bowl and add the soup. If desired, soup can be strained.

Potato soup
½ leek, cut into thin strips
½ carrot, sliced
½ tbs wholemeal flour
5 dl vegetable broth
1 medium-sized potato, diced
Small amount of miso
Basil, marjoram
1 tbs cream

Sauté the leek and carrot in a small amount of vegetable broth. Sprinkle with wholemeal flour and add the vegetable broth. Add potato and cook until soft. Season to taste. Place basil, marjoram and optional cream in the soup bowl, and add the finished soup.

Minestrone*
½ tbs health food store vegetable fat
2 tbs leek
Small amount of onion, finely chopped
A few celery (celeriac) leaves
½ plate mangold leaves
7 dl water or vegetable broth
1 tbs lovage or thyme
½ garlic clove, pressed
Basil, parsley, chives
15 g wholegrain pasta or wholegrain rice
5 g butter, vegetable margarine
or nut spread

Mince onion, leek, celery (celeriac) leaves and mangold leaves, and sauté slowly. Add vegetable broth, season and cook for 30 minutes. Add pasta or rice and cook another 15–20 minutes. To enhance flavour, add nut spread or vegetable margarine.

* Omit if on a strict sodium-free diet.

Vegetables

Spinach, chopped*
¼ l vegetable broth
200 g spinach (remove thick stems)
¼ garlic clove, pressed
Peppermint leaves, sage
1 cup raw spinach
Fresh butter or vegetable health food store
margarine (optional)

Briefly cook spinach in the vegetable broth and drain, then cut, chop or blend. Return spinach to the pan and heat. Add garlic and herbs. Chop or blend the raw spinach, and add fresh butter or vegetable margarine before serving.

* Omit if on a strict no-salt diet.

Spinach, whole leaves*
300 g spinach (remove thick stems, briefly boil the coarser winter spinach if required)
1 tbs pine nuts
1 tbs raisins (optional)
Peppermint leaves, sage, parsley
Melted butter or health food store vegetable margarine (optional)

Sauté spinach uncovered over low heat with a small amount of water. Add pine nuts, spices and raisins (optional), and continue cooking briefly. Add melted butter or vegetable margarine (optional).

* Omit if on a strict no-salt diet.

Romaine lettuce*
1 romaine lettuce
1 l water
Small amount of chopped onion
½ tbs health food store vegetable fat
1 dl vegetable broth
2 tbs cream

Halve the romaine lettuce, boil until medium-soft then drain. Reassemble the lettuce and place in an ovenproof baking dish. Lightly sauté the onion with vegetable fat and sprinkle over the lettuce. Add vegetable broth and cook in the oven for 30–40 minutes. Pour cream over the mixture 5 minutes before serving.

* Omit if on a strict no-salt diet.

Endive/chicory*
1 large head of chicory/endive

Prepared like romaine lettuce.

* Omit if on a strict sodium-free diet.

Sautéed chicory/endive
2 stalks of chicory/endive
½ tbs health food store vegetable fat
3 tbs vegetable broth
Marjoram, thyme
Small amount of butter or vegetable margarine or nut spread

Halve the chicory/endive stalks and layer them in the pan. Add heated vegetable fat and vegetable broth to the chicory/endive. Season and simmer covered over low heat for 30 minutes. Spread melted butter, vegetable margarine or nut spread on the prepared vegetable.

Swiss chard with béchamel sauce
3 branches of Swiss chard
½ tbs health food store vegetable fat
½ dl vegetable broth
Small amount of lemon juice or
1 tsp almond puree
Estragon, parsley and chives
Béchamel sauce (see recipe page 59)

Sauté the Swiss chard cut into pieces 3 cm long in vegetable fat, add the vegetable broth with lemon juice or almond puree, and cook covered over low heat for 30–45 minutes until soft. Season. Add béchamel sauce to the cooked vegetables.

Swiss chard or false asparagus
3–4 branches of Swiss chard
½ tbs health food store vegetable fat
½ small onion
2 tbs milk or a small amount of lemon juice
1 dl vegetable broth
Estragon, bay leaf, clove, parsley, chive
Remoulade sauce (see recipe page 60)

Place in the pan the prepared Swiss chard cut 10 cm long. Place the onions sautéed in health food margarine over the branches, add milk or lemon juice and vegetable broth, and cook over low heat for 30–45 minutes until tender. Serve with remoulade sauce or melt the Swiss chards with grated salt-free cheese and a small amount of hot butter.

Celery stalks*
3–4 celery stalks
½ onion, chopped
Small amount of apple, finely chopped
1 dl vegetable broth
1 tsp almond puree
Small amount of Kelpamare
Celery root (celeriac) with stalks and leaves

Cut the celery stalks into pieces 8 cm long and place in a pan. Briefly sauté the onion and apple without fat and spread on the celery stalks. Add vegetable broth and almond puree and cook over low heat for 30–45 minutes until soft. Season to taste.

* Omit if on a strict sodium-free diet.

Baked fennel with cream cheese crème
1 large or 2 small fennel plants
Pepper
Several drops of lemon juice
Small amount of cream cheese

Quarter the fennel and steam it until fairly soft. Pull apart the individual layers of the fennel bulb and place them in an ovenproof mould. Drizzle with lemon juice. Stir the cream cheese with 2 tbs of fennel stock and spread over the vegetables. Bake in hot oven.

Vegetable curry
1 tbs olive oil
1 spring onion
200 g vegetables (e.g. leeks, carrots, courgettes, asparagus)
½ tsp wholemeal flour
Pinch of curry powder
½ tsp vegetable broth
½ orange
1 tsp sultanas
Pinch of whole cane sugar (or Succanat)
Small amount of pepper

Slice the spring onion into fine rings and cook in slightly heated oil. Sprinkle in flour and curry powder, and add the vegetable broth. Add the finely cut vegetables and cook covered for approx. 15 minutes. Set aside two or three wedges of the orange, squeeze the rest and place the sultanas in the juice. When the vegetables are soft, add the sultanas and orange juice, heat the mixture and season with sugar and a small amount of pepper. Serve and spread the orange wedges on top.

Cooked carrots
3–4 carrots
1 dl vegetable broth
1 tsp almond puree
1 pinch of fruit sugar
Marjoram, thyme, rosemary, parsley

Cut the carrots in strips or rounds and sauté in the vegetable broth for 30–45 minutes. Stir in the almond puree (optional). Season to taste. Sprinkle with chopped parsley.

Peas and carrots
½ tbs health food store vegetable fat
100 g fresh sweet peas, shelled
1 dl vegetable broth
Marjoram, thyme, lovage, parsley, chives
150 g sliced carrots, prepared according to the recipe for cooked carrots

Briefly sauté peas in the health food store vegetable fat, add vegetable broth and cook until soft. Season to taste. Mix carrots and peas, or serve them separately on the platter.

Peas, French style
¼ head of lettuce or romaine lettuce
150–200 g peas, shelled
1 dl vegetable broth
Parsley, chives, marjoram, thyme, lovage
10 g nut spread
1 tsp wholemeal flour

Sauté the lettuce or romaine lettuce (cut into fine strips) with the peas in the vegetable broth over very low heat until soft. Season to taste. Mix nut spread with wholemeal flour, add and boil briefly.

Cooked sugar peas (snow peas)
200 g sugar peas
1 dl vegetable broth
1 pinch sugar (Succanat)
Small amount of parsley or lovage, chives, marjoram, thyme
Fresh butter, vegetable margarine or nut spread

Cook sugar peas and herbs covered in the vegetable broth for 30–45 minutes. Season and add fresh butter, vegetable margarine or nut spread when serving.

Green beans with tomatoes
½ health food store margarine
½ onion
250 g beans
Small amount of garlic
Savory, parsley
1–2 tomatoes
Small amount of caraway, marjoram, lovage

Sauté chopped onion in health food store margarine. Add and steam the beans, finely diced tomatoes and herbs for approx. 1 hour. Add water if necessary. Season to taste.

Celery root (celeriac), sautéed*
½ health food store margarine
½ onion
½ celery root (celeriac)
1 dl vegetable broth
Small amount of lemon juice, marjoram
1 tsp almond puree
Very thin slices of apple, nuts

Sauté the chopped onions in health food store margarine. Pour the vegetable broth over the celery root (celeriac) cut in rectangular slices and cook for 30–45 minutes until soft. Season to taste. To refine, add almond puree and, if desired, apple slices. Sprinkle with chopped nuts.

* Omit if on a strict sodium-free diet.

Celery root (celeriac) with béchamel sauce*
Prepare one 1 small celery root (celeriac) as described above and mix with béchamel sauce (see recipe page 59).

* Omit if on a strict sodium-free diet.

Black salsify, sautéed
Approx. 250 g black salsify (cleaned and prepared)
½ tbs health food store vegetable fat
½ onion
½ dl milk
1 dl vegetable broth
Lemon, lovage, bay leaf, clove, basil
Small amount of miso
Parsley, chives

Cut salsify into finger-length pieces and put into pan. Add the chopped onion sautéed in vegetable fat, milk and vegetable broth, season and cook over low heat for 1 hour. Sprinkle fresh parsley and chive when serving.

Beetroot (red beet)
Cut off the root tips and leaves to approx. 2 cm, and wash thoroughly without damaging the skin.

350 g beetroot (red beet)
1 dl vegetable broth
Pinch of fruit sugar
¼ laurel leaf, lovage, caraway, nutmeg
Very small amount of garlic, parsley
Small amount of lemon juice, lemon balm
1 tbs wholemeal flour, mixed with cold water
1 tbs almond puree

Cook the beetroots (red beets) in pressure cooker until soft, about 25 minutes. Peel then cut into fine slices. Mix thoroughly in the vegetable broth with the herbs and spices, and cook over low heat for 15 minutes. Stir in the wholemeal flour and add the almond puree to bind.

Jerusalem artichoke
250 g Jerusalem artichoke
Small amount of vegetable broth
Basil
1 tsp almond puree

Cook the Jerusalem artichoke like bouillon potatoes (see recipe page 52). Peel, slice and cook in the vegetable broth until soft. Season and add the almond puree to refine.
You can also prepare the Jerusalem artichoke with béchamel sauce (see recipe page 59) and grated cheese.

Tomatoes, stewed
4–5 tomatoes
½ tbs health food store vegetable fat
½ onion
Fruit sugar
Touch of garlic
Rosemary, marjoram, basil
1 tbs cornflour (optional)
Parsley or chives or dill

Slightly brown onion and fruit sugar in vegetable fat in the pan. Douse the tomatoes with boiling water then peel, cut into pieces, add to the onion and cook the mixture until it begins to thicken. Add garlic and spices, and finish cooking (add cornflour to thicken). Generously sprinkle chopped parsley or other herbs on the prepared tomatoes.

Tomatoes, baked
2–3 tomatoes
10 g health food store vegetable fat or butter
½ onion, chopped
Pinch of herbes de Provence (basil, rosemary, thyme, sage) and parsley

Sauté the onion without vegetable fat. Put the halved tomatoes on a greased tray or ovenproof mould. Place dabs of vegetable fat, butter or olive oil onto each tomato half, then spread the sautéed onion and herbs over them. Cook briefly in the oven.
Other tomatoes may be blended or very finely chopped, mixed with cream, heated quickly and spread over the prepared tomatoes.

Tomatoes with cheese slices
2 tomatoes
30 g salt-free cheese
Parsley

Cut tomatoes in half and place on a greased baking tray or in an ovenproof mould. Cut the cheese into thin slices the size of the tomatoes and place a slice on each half. Bake in the oven until the cheese is melted. Sprinkle with parsley.

Tomatoes, stuffed
2–3 tomatoes
1 tsp rice per tomato
Butter or vegetable margarine or nut spread
Small amount of onion and garlic, rosemary, marjoram, thyme, basil, bay leaf, nutmeg
Vegetable broth (optional)

Cut off the tops of the tomatoes and hollow out the core. Chop the tomato pulp and mix with 1 tsp uncooked rice and the herbs and spices. Fill in the core with the mixture, add dabs of butter or vegetable margarine or nut spread, and put back the tops on the tomatoes. Bake in the oven at a high bottom heat for 20–30 minutes.

Tomatoes à la provençale
2 tomatoes
1 tbs chopped parsley
1 tbs breadcrumbs

Halve tomatoes and place on a tray. Mix breadcrumbs and parsley, and spread over the tomatoes with a spoon. Bake in the oven for 15 minutes.

Courgette and tomato medley
½ tbs health food store vegetable fat
½ onion, chopped
300 g courgette
50 g tomato
Garlic, rosemary, marjoram, thyme, basil, parsley, chive, dill
Small amount of cornflour (optional)
1 tsp almond puree

Lightly sauté the onion with vegetable fat. Dice the courgettes. Peel and dice tomatoes. Add the vegetables to the onions and cook until soft. Season to taste. If too liquid, add stirred cornflour and 1 tsp almond puree before serving.

Recipes Sweet peppers (green, yellow, red)
These are very suitable as an addition to other dishes.
150–200 g sweet peppers
½ tbs health food store vegetable fat
½ onion, chopped
Garlic, rosemary, marjoram, thyme, basil, parsley

Cut the sweet peppers in strips and sauté them in vegetable fat with the onion, herbs and spices in a covered pan for 30 minutes.

Ratatouille
50 g sweet pepper
100 g courgette
50 g aubergine
1 tomato
½ onion, chopped
Small amount of garlic
1 tbs health food store vegetable fat
Rosemary, marjoram, thyme, basil, parsley

Dice the sweet peppers, courgettes, aubergines and tomato (peeled). Sauté onion and garlic in the vegetable fat, add vegetables and cook covered for 1 hour. Season to taste. If there is too much sauce, leave to thicken while uncovered.

Aubergines (eggplant)
400–500 g aubergines
1 tbs health food store vegetable fat
Small amount of vegetable broth (optional)
Small amount of Kelpamare
1–2 tomatoes

Wash the aubergines, peel if necessary, and sauté the cubed aubergines in vegetable fat until soft. Season with a small amount of Kelpamare. Garnish with a few tomato halves or stewed tomatoes.

Artichokes
1 artichoke
¾ l water
1 tbs lemon juice
Pinch of sea salt (optional)
Yoghurt dressing (see recipe page 33)

Cut off the stalks close to the artichokes. Remove the bottommost hard leaves and tips. Halve and cut out the heart, rinse under running water and rub the cut surface with lemon juice. Boil water, add lemon juice and sea salt and cook the artichoke until soft for approx. 45 minutes. Drain and serve the artichoke on a warm platter covered with a serviette. Serve with yoghurt dressing.

Asparagus
½ bunch asparagus
1 l water
Pinch of sea salt
Grated, salt-free cheese
Nut spread

Wash the asparagus and carefully peel the stalks. Green asparagus can be left almost whole. Cook the asparagus in boiling water until soft for 20–30 minutes (green asparagus take much less time), remove with a slotted spoon and serve on a platter covered with a serviette. Sprinkle grated cheese and pour liquid nut spread over the dish.
As a variation, serve with vinaigrette (see recipe page 60).

Cauliflower or broccoli
Organic only.
1 small cauliflower or broccoli (250 g)
1 tsp health food store vegetable fat
1 garlic clove
1 dl vegetable broth
Small amount of pepper
Pine nuts or almond slices

Cut off the leaves and stalk below the florets. Peel the stalk and cut into larger pieces; divide the flower into florets. Lightly brown the chopped garlic clove in vegetable fat, add the cauliflower or broccoli, and sauté briefly. Cover with the vegetable broth and then simmer for approx. 5 minutes. Season with pepper. Briefly warm pine nuts or sliced almond in a pan (without fat) and sprinkle over the vegetables.

You can also mix the vegetables with a béchamel sauce (see recipe page 59). Alternatively, serve à la polonaise: mix ½ hard-boiled egg, finely chopped, a little parsley, ½ tbs of grated salt-free cheese with 1 tbs of hot (not brown) butter and spread over the vegetables.

Kohlrabi with herbs
1 kohlrabi
1 dl vegetable broth
1 tbs tender kohlrabi leaves, chopped
1 tbs cream
Béchamel sauce (see recipe page 59)

Quarter the kohlrabi then cut into fine slices. Cook covered in the vegetable broth for 30–45 minutes. Add the kohlrabi leaves and cream before serving. Mix the béchamel sauce with chopped herbs and pour over the cooked kohlrabi.

Brussels sprouts, sautéed
½ tbs health food store vegetable fat
200 g Brussels sprouts, cleaned
1 dl vegetable broth
Nutmeg, basil

Briefly sauté Brussels sprouts in vegetable fat. Add vegetable broth and continue cooking for 30 minutes until soft. Season to taste.
Add a small amount of melted butter when serving (optional).

Cabbage or white cabbage, sautéed
Avoid if suffering from meteorism. All cabbage types must be carefully chewed, and raw cabbage juice is always permitted.
½ tbs health food store vegetable fat
½ onion, chopped
250 g young cabbage
1 dl vegetable broth
Small amount of Kelpamare (optional)
Nutmeg, caraway, pinch of sea salt, basil or lovage

Sauté onions in vegetable fat, add cabbage cut in strips 2 cm wide and cook until the vegetables begin to soften. Add vegetable broth and cook over low heat for 30 minutes until soft. Season to taste.

Green, mature cabbage must be blanched briefly before cooking.

Cabbage, chopped
Avoid if suffering from meteorism.
200 g cabbage
1 l water
½ tbs health food store vegetable fat
Hint of garlic
1 small tbs flour
1 dl vegetable broth or half milk, half vegetable broth
1–2 tbs cream
Small amount of Kelpamare, nutmeg, caraway, parsley

Cut the cabbage into 4 pieces, steam until soft, drain and mince. Sauté briefly in vegetable fat, sprinkle with finely chopped garlic and flour, and cook for 15 minutes. Add vegetable broth or milk and heat. Season to taste. Enrich with cream.

Colewort
Prepare like cabbage.

Red cabbage
Avoid if suffering from meteorism.
½ tbs health food store vegetable fat
250 g red cabbage
½ tbs lemon juice
½ apple
½ tbs rice
1 dl vegetable broth
½ dl grape or apple juice
1 apple
Small amount of butter

Sauté the finely grated red cabbage in vegetable fat. Add lemon juice, finely sliced apple and rice. Continue sautéing. Add vegetable broth and grape juice (or apple juice) and cook covered over low heat until soft, for 1–1½ hours. Peel the second apple and cut into wedges. Baste with butter and braise the apple wedges on a tin in the oven. Garnish the prepared red cabbage with the apple wedges.

Leeks
Avoid if suffering from meteorism.
200 g leek, cleaned and prepared
½ tbs health food store vegetable fat
1 dl vegetable broth
½ tbs cream
Small amount of grated salt-free cheese (optional)

Cut leeks into 10 cm pieces and layer them in the pan. Add vegetable fat and vegetable broth, and cook covered slowly. After cooking, add cream and sprinkle with grated cheese (optional).

Chestnut vegetables
250 g chestnuts
½ tbs health food store vegetable fat
½ tbs fruit sugar or Succanat
1 dl vegetable broth
1 tbs cream
Fresh butter

Score the chestnuts and place them in the hot oven. Peel them. Roast the fructose or Succanat in the health food store margarine until brown and drench with vegetable broth. Add the chestnuts and cook for about 30 minutes until the liquid has evaporated. Spread fresh butter over the chestnuts. You can also prepare the chestnuts without sugar: Sauté the prepared chestnuts with a chopped onion and finish cooking with stock. Spread a steamed onion cut into strips over the arranged chestnuts.

Lentils
150 g lentils
2 dl vegetable broth
1 studded onion
½ tbs health food store vegetable fat
½ onion
½ tbs lemon juice or 1 tbs cream

Soak lentils overnight and drain. Cook the lentils in the vegetable broth with the onion until soft. Sauté the chopped onion in the vegetable fat, sprinkle the flour and add to the lentils. Enhance with lemon juice or cream. Some types of lentils (e.g. red lentils) do not need to be soaked and have a short cooking time.

Salads of Cooked Vegetables

Carrots, celery root (celeriac), beetroot (red beet), beans, cauliflower, broccoli, courgettes, mangold leaves and Swiss chard are particularly suitable for these salads.
Cook the vegetables in vegetable broth or water until soft. Drain and dice or slice into florets or strips.
Serve with salad dressing, vinaigrette or mayonnaise. Enhance with onions and chopped herbs.

Potato salad
200 g potatoes
½ dl vegetable broth
1 tbs mayonnaise (see recipe page 60)
½ tbs onions, chopped
Borage, chives, parsley,
lemon balm, marjoram, thyme, dill

Cook the potatoes in the pressure cooker until soft, peel while hot and slice. Pour the heated vegetable broth and let stand for a few minutes, then mix in the mayonnaise. Season with onions and herbs. Mayonnaise can be replaced with oil, lemon juice and cream, well mixed and added to the potatoes.

Potato salad with cucumbers
1 large potato
¼ cucumber
2 tbs yoghurt dressing (see recipe page 33)
½ garlic clove
Dill or borage, chives,
parsley, onion

Prepare the potato as described above. Grate the peeled cucumber with a coarse grater and add to the potato. Mix with

yoghurt dressing and season with onions and herbs.
Rub the salad bowl with the garlic clove before serving.

Salade niçoise*
1 boiled potato
1 small tomato
Radishes
Several cucumber slices
1 hard-boiled egg
1 tbs oil
½ tbs lemon juice
Parsley, chives or dill,
lemon balm, borage
A few leaves of head lettuce

Slice the potato, tomato, radishes and egg. Add to the cucumber slices and mix with a salad dressing of oil, lemon juice and herbs. Just before serving, cut the leaves of head lettuce into broad strips and mix with the salad, or prepare the salad on the lettuce leaves.

* Omit if on a strict sodium-free diet.

Rice salad
50 g rice
2 dl water
2 tbs quark dressing (see recipe page 34)
½ tbs onion, chopped
¼ tomato
Chives, parsley or basil
A few salad leaves

Cook the rice in water, rinse briefly and let cool. Add onions, finely diced tomato and herbs to the quark dressing.
Mix the rice with the dressing and prepare on salad leaves.

Celery root (celeriac) salad* with soy mayonnaise
½ small celery root (celeriac)
½–1 tbs lemon juice
2 walnuts
¼ apple (optional)
1 tbs soy mayonnaise (see recipe page 34)

Grate or cut the raw celery root (celeriac) into match-thin strips. Add lemon juice to prevent browning. Add the coarsely chopped walnuts and the grated apple, and mix with the mayonnaise.

* Omit if on a strict sodium-free diet.

Vegetable aspic
2½ dl vegetable broth
2 g agar-agar
A few drops of lemon juice
Small amount of Kelpamare
Fresh cucumber slices
Tomato, diced
Broccoli flowers, cooked
Peas, cooked
Beans, cooked and finely chopped

Agar-agar is a plant-based gelatine powder that is used for vegetable and fruit aspics, sauces, puddings, etc. instead of animal gelatine.
Add agar-agar powder to the lukewarm vegetable broth and heat slowly until the gelling agent is thoroughly dissolved. Season with lemon juice and Kelpamare. Pour a small amount of aspic into the rinsed moulds and let harden. Garnish with vegetable slices, add more aspic, leave to harden and repeat until the moulds are filled.
Turn over the cooled aspics and serve on salad leaves.

Potato Dishes

Potatoes in their skins
Low-starch potatoes are particularly suitable.
3–4 small potatoes
Water

Brush and wash potatoes. Fill pan with steamer insert or wire screen with water up to the insert, add potatoes, cover and cook for 30–40 minutes (8–10 minutes in the pressure cooker).

Baked potatoes (in their jackets)
3–4 small potatoes
1 tbs oil
Butter or nut spread

Brush and wash the potatoes. Score the peel on the top 3–4 times, brush with oil and bake the potatoes on a greased tray at medium heat for 30–40 minutes. Dab nut spread on each of the cooked potatoes.

Quark potatoes
3–4 small potatoes
50 g low-fat quark
1–2 tbs milk or cream
Chives, caraway or marjoram
Pinch of rock salt

Make a shallow cut into the top of the potatoes and prepare them as for baked (jacket) potatoes. For the stuffing, stir quark with milk or cream until smooth, then add seasonings. Use a spoon to spread into the shallow cut of the baked (jacket) potatoes or apply with a piping bag.

Caraway potatoes
2–3 medium-sized, longish narrow potatoes
1 tsp caraway
1 tbs olive oil

Wash and clean the potatoes and cut them crosswise in half. Sprinkle caraway on the cut side. Place the potatoes cut side down on a greased tray, brush with olive oil and bake at medium heat for 45 minutes.

Bouillon potatoes
250 g potatoes
1–2 dl vegetable broth
Lovage, thyme
10 g butter or vegetable margarine or nut spread

Wash potatoes then peel, halve or cut them into pieces and cook until soft in the vegetable broth with the spices. Spread butter, vegetable margarine or nut spread on the prepared potatoes.

Cream potatoes
200 g potatoes
Onion, chopped
1 dl vegetable broth
½ dl cream or milk (optional)
Thyme, nutmeg,
parsley

Peel, slice and briefly sauté (without vegetable fat) the potatoes and onion. Add the vegetable broth and spices, and cook until soft. Add cream or milk before serving. Sprinkle the prepared potatoes with chopped parsley.

Potatoes with tomatoes
200 g potatoes
½ small onion
1 dl vegetable broth
1 small tomato
1 tbs cream or sesame cream (see recipe page 38)
Marjoram, rosemary or thyme

Briefly sauté (without fat) the chopped onion and peeled, sliced potatoes, then cook them in the vegetable broth until medium-soft. Cut the peeled tomato into wedges, add and finish cooking. Season to taste. Add the cream or sesame cream before serving.

Potato mash
4 potatoes
Water
Dried tomatoes
Butter, vegetable margarine or nut spread

Wash, peel, slice and steam the potatoes until soft. Pass directly through a potato press onto a warm platter. Add melted butter, vegetable margarine or nut spread, and garnish with minced dried tomatoes.

Potato puree
4 potatoes
Small amount of water
1 dl milk
Nutmeg
1 tbs cream (optional)
Marjoram and caraway, finely chopped
Hint of garlic
Dried tomatoes

Peel the potatoes, cut in pieces, steam until soft. Pass through a potato press. Heat milk, add the potato puree, stir until smooth and season. Add cream if desired. Serve on a hot platter, garnished with finely cut dried tomatoes or with onion rings roasted until golden yellow.

Potato dumplings
4 potatoes
1 dl milk
10 g butter
10 g butter or nut spread
Nutmeg

Prepare potatoes as for potato puree, season with nutmeg. Dip a small ladle in the melted butter, cut out dumplings and serve on hot platter. Dress with butter or nut spread.

Potato cakes
2 potatoes
Small amount of water
1 egg
Roasted onions
Small amount of flour
Health food store vegetable fat or oil

Steam the peeled potatoes until soft and strain. Mix with the egg and the roasted onions. Shape small cakes with a little flour and bake them half-floating in oil or vegetable fat on both sides.

Roast potatoes
2 small potatoes
Small amount of water
1 dl vegetable broth
1–2 tbs cream, sesame cream (see recipe page 38) or nut spread
Nutmeg, thyme,
parsley

Peel and halve potatoes and steam them until medium-soft. Put them on an oven-proof platter with the cut side down. Cover with vegetable broth. Season and roast in the oven until the liquid has thickened. Add cream or nut spread and continue roasting until the potatoes are lightly browned. Serve with the cut side facing up and sprinkle with chopped parsley.

Princess potatoes
3 potatoes
Small amount of water
1 tbs salt-free cheese or quark
½ tbs health food store vegetable fat
1 dl milk
1 egg
2 tbs milk
1 tbs cream, or sesame cream
Pieces of butter
Nutmeg, finely chopped marjoram

Steam the potatoes, peel and cut into thick slices. Place them in an ovenproof mould and mix in the grated cheese or curd. Season. Pour over the vegetable fat and milk, and bake in the oven for 10 minutes. Mix the beaten egg with milk and cream and pour over the top. Spread the pieces of butter on top and bake the potatoes in the oven for 10–15 minutes.

Lyonnaise potatoes
1 tbs health food store margarine
½ tbs oil
3 small potatoes
1 small onion

Heat health food store margarine or oil. Cook the peeled, sliced potatoes in the hot fat until they soften. Add the onion cut into strips and finish cooking.

Potato chips (cooked raw)
3 large potatoes
½ tbs health food store margarine or
½ tbs olive oil
Nutmeg, rosemary

Peel the potatoes, cut into chips and dry in a towel. Heat margarine or oil and add the chips. Cook shortly covered and then for 30 minutes uncovered. Season to taste.

Potato goulash
1 onion
1 large potato
1 green sweet pepper
1–2 dl water
Marjoram, thyme, rosemary, parsley

Finely dice the onion and potato, julienne the sweet pepper and cover with water in a pan. Cook until soft, approx. 15 minutes. Season well and serve.

Potatoes with kale (stew)
½ health food store margarine
1 tbs onion, chopped
100 g kale
2 small potatoes
Small amount of hot butter
Finely chopped caraway, marjoram, nutmeg

Sauté the onion in the margarine and add the finely chopped spring cabbage. Add the peeled, diced potatoes and cook for 30–45 minutes. Season. Pour a little hot butter over the potatoes.

Ayurveda potatoes
This attractive, aromatic dish yields 3–4 helpings.
5 large potatoes
½ soy drink
1 package of soy crème (substitute for crème fraîche)
1 bunch each of fresh dill, chives and parsley
Juice of ½ lemon
1–2 tsp turmeric
½ tsp curry
Dash of soya sauce (optional)

Cut the thoroughly cleaned potatoes into thick slices and cook them for approx. 5 minutes. Meanwhile slowly heat the soy drink in a pan, mixed with the soy crème (do not boil). Stir in turmeric to taste, add curry then season with soy sauce. Put the potato slices in the sauce and simmer for approx. 10 minutes. Sprinkle the fresh, finely chopped herbs on the potatoes and serve at once.

Grain Dishes

Japanese rice
80 g wholegrain rice
1–2 dl vegetable stock
10 g butter or vegetable margarine or nut spread
1 small peeled onion studded with clove, and bay leaf

Put the rice in the cooking stock with the studded onion and boil for 40 minutes. Leave to cool and remove the onion. Reheat the rice in the oven and top with heated butter, vegetable margarine or nut spread before serving.

Risotto
80 g wholegrain rice
½ tbs health food store margarine
1 tbs onion, chopped
2 dl vegetable broth or water
Dried mushrooms
Fresh herbs, to taste
Rosemary
10 g fresh butter,
vegetable margarine or nut spread

Sauté onion in the margarine, add rice and sauté until translucent. Add the vegetable broth or hot water and cook until al dente (30–40 minutes). Add the finely chopped dried mushrooms and herbs, and cook briefly together. Before serving, mix in butter, vegetable margarine or nut spread with a fork.

Saffron rice
Prepare like risotto. Dissolve a pinch of saffron powder in a small amount of stock and add to rice.

Riz creole with vegetables
½ tbs health food store vegetable fat
80 g wholegrain rice
2 tbs vegetables, e.g. leeks, celery root (celeriac), carrots, finely diced
2 dl vegetable broth
Freshly chopped herbs, to taste

Briefly sauté rice and vegetables, add hot vegetable broth and herbs, and cook for 30–45 minutes.

* Omit if on a strict sodium-free diet.

Tomato rice
80 g wholegrain rice
½ health food store margarine
1 tbs onion, chopped
Small amount of garlic, pressed
1 large tomato
Approx. 1 dl vegetable broth
Rosemary, marjoram, nutmeg
Basil (optional)
Pinch of whole cane sugar (Succanat)
10 g butter or vegetable margarine

Sauté onion and garlic in the margarine, add rice and sauté until translucent. Add peeled, diced tomato. Add vegetable broth and spices, then cook for 30–45 minutes. Add fresh butter or vegetable margarine before serving.

Rice with courgettes
½ tbs health food store vegetable fat
80 g wholegrain rice
1 tbs onion, chopped
150 g tender courgettes
1½ dl vegetable broth or water
Freshly chopped dill
10 g butter or vegetable margarine or nut spread

Dice the courgettes. Prepare dish as for tomato rice (see above).

Rice with spinach*
80 g wholegrain rice
½ health food store margarine
100 g spinach
Small amount of chopped onion
2 dl vegetable broth or water
Nutmeg and peppermint
10 g fresh butter or vegetable margarine or nut spread

Cut spinach coarsely. Prepare dish further as for tomato rice (see recipe page 55).

* Omit if on a strict sodium-free diet.

Rice with peas (risi e bisi)
80 g wholegrain rice
150 g fresh young peas, shelled
½ health food store margarine
Small amount of chopped onion
Pinch each of fruit sugar and sea salt
½ dl vegetable broth
Small amount of chopped onion
1½–2 dl water
10 g butter or vegetable margarine or nut spread
Parsley

Sauté onion with fruit sugar and sea salt in margarine. Add the peas and cook briefly, then add vegetable broth and cook the peas until soft. Prepare risotto (see recipe page 54) in a separate pan. Add the cooked peas. Before serving, top the prepared rice with butter, vegetable margarine or nut spread and chopped parsley.

Rice gratin with tomatoes
½ tbs health food store vegetable fat
80 g wholegrain rice
2 small tomatoes
Small amount of chopped onion

2 tbs vegetables, e.g. leeks, celery root (celeriac)*, carrots
1 ½ dl vegetable broth
1 tbs sea salt
Parsley, lovage
10 g butter or vegetable margarine

Briefly sauté onion and very finely diced vegetables, add the rice and continue cooking until translucent. Cover with hot vegetable broth, then season and cook for 30–45 minutes. Layer the finished rice and the sliced tomatoes in an ovenproof mould, top with dabs of butter or vegetable margarine, and bake in the oven for 10 minutes.

* Omit if on a strict sodium-free diet.

Indian rice dish
80 g wholegrain rice
2 dl vegetable broth
1 small banana
1 small apple
1 tbs raisins
1 tsp sunflower seeds
1 tsp sesame seeds
Saffron, curry, fresh ginger root

Cook rice with vegetable broth until not quite soft (approx. 30–40 minutes). Mix the sliced banana, the peeled and thinly sliced apple, and the raisins into the rice and continue cooking for 5–10 minutes. Season with saffron, curry and ginger root to taste. Sprinkle with sunflower seeds and lightly dry-roasted (without fat) sesame seeds.

Semolina mash
50 g semolina
3 dl milk
2 dl water
1 tbs sesame cream (see recipe page 38)
1 tbs each of fruit sugar and cinnamon

Stir semolina into the boiling liquid and cook for 15–20 minutes. Sprinkle the cream and fruit sugar mixed with cinnamon onto the prepared semolina mash.

Semolina gnocchi
50 g semolina
Approx. 3 dl vegetable broth
Nutmeg
1 egg
½ dl milk
2 tbs cream
1 tbs chives
1 tbs salt-free cheese
10 g butter

Stir semolina into the boiling milk, season with nutmeg and cook for 15–20 minutes. Spread about 1 ½ cm thick on a board, let cool and cut out round cookies. First place the leftover pieces in a buttered baking dish and then arrange the round cookies nicely on top. Whisk the egg with the milk and cream, and pour it on top; sprinkle with chives, grated cheese and butter flakes. Bake slowly in the oven until the egg mixture is firm.

Polenta
½ tbs olive oil
50 g maize semolina, medium fine
3 dl water
Nutmeg
½ tbs fresh butter or
vegetable margarine or nut spread

Oil the pan. Boil water and stir in the maize. Cook for 5 minutes over low heat, stirring frequently. Season and continue cooking for 45–60 minutes over low heat. Add butter, vegetable margarine or nut spread before serving. You may also add onion slices sautéed without fat.

Polenta slices
50 g maize
20 g semolina
3 ½ dl water
1 tsp health food store vegetable fat
Nutmeg
Chives, parsley or basil

Process maize, semolina and water into polenta, season to taste. Spread hot polenta 1 ½ cm thick on a board and leave to cool. Cut in squares and cook them to a golden yellow in heated vegetable fat.

Millet risotto
½ tbs health food store vegetable fat
50 g millet
1 tbs onion, chopped
1 ½ dl vegetable broth
½ onion

Sauté onion and hot-rinsed millet in vegetable fat until glazed. Add hot vegetable broth, and boil for 20 minutes. When serving, add onion slices or rings roasted without fat.

Millet risotto with vegetables
40 g millet
1 tbs onion, chopped
2 tbs diced vegetable
(leek, celery root (celeriac)*, carrots or carrots with peas)
1 ½ dl vegetable broth
Small amount of Kelpamare (optional)
Rosemary
1 tbs grated salt-free cheese (optional)
10 g fresh butter or nut spread

Sauté onion, diced vegetable and millet rinsed hot until glazed. Add hot vegetable broth, season and boil for 20 minutes. When serving, top with grated cheese (optional) and dabs of butter or nut spread.

* Omit if on a strict sodium-free diet.

Coarse-ground grain mash
2 tbs coarse-ground grain (wheat, oats, rye)
3 tbs water

Soak the coarse-ground grain for 12 hours. Using the same water, boil for 10 minutes or cook for 1 hour in a bain-marie.

Noodles, spaghetti, macaroni etc.
For a strict healing diet, egg pasta should not be used. Today high-quality wholegrain, soy and spelt pastas can be easily found in addition to well-known Italian pasta products made from wheat. Note that many sauces contain large amounts of fat (oil, butter, cheese, cream).
The best-tolerated pasta products are cooked al dente with a classic or simple tomato sauce (see recipes in chapter on sauces).

Spätzle or Knöpfli (without egg)
60 g wholemeal flour
20 g soy flour
1 dl diluted milk
1 l water
1 tbs health food store vegetable margarine
Onion, julienned
Chives and parsley

Mix wholemeal and soy flour thoroughly with diluted milk and tap the mixture until the dough forms bubbles. Let rest for at least 1 hour.
Boil water. Press the dough in portions through a coarse screen into the boiling water or place it onto a small wooden cutting board, cut fine strips with a knife and drop them into the boiling water. Let the Knöpfli or Spätzle simmer until they rise to the surface. Remove with a skimmer and place on a hot platter. As desired, garnish with julienned onion sautéed in vegetable fat (or without fat), chives and parsley.

Spinach* or tomato Knöpfli
70 g wholemeal flour (of which $1/3$ soy flour)
1 egg
1 dl diluted milk
1 handful of chopped, raw spinach or 1 tsp tomato puree
1 dl water
Chives and parsley

Make a smooth batter from the wholemeal, soy flour, egg and water, and let rest for 1 hour. Add spinach or tomato puree. Season with chives and parsley. Then prepare and cook Knöpfli or Spätzle, according to the recipe page 57.

* Omit if on a strict sodium-free diet.

Oat flake dumplings
½ health food store margarine
1 tbs chopped onion
2 tbs finely cut leek, celery root (celeriac)*, spinach
50 g oat flakes
½ dl vegetable broth
Vegetable margarine or sunflower oil
Peppermint or savage

Sauté onion and vegetables in the margarine, add oat flakes and vegetable broth and cook to a thick mash. Season to taste. Spread mash 1 cm thick on a board and leave to cool. Cut rectangles. Heat margarine or oil and cook dumplings until golden yellow on both sides.

* Omit if on a strict sodium-free diet.

Omelette
50 g flour
1 egg
1 dl diluted milk
Small amount of health food store vegetable fat

Sift the flour into a bowl, add the egg and slowly add the liquid, beating vigorously. The batter should flow from the ladle in a thread. Leave for at least 1 hour. Heat the vegetable fat, pour in a little batter for the thinnest possible omelettes. Bake to a golden brown colour on both sides over medium-high heat.

French omelette
2 eggs
2 tbs milk
Nutmeg
1 tbs chopped herbs (chives, parsley, rosemary, basil, marjoram)
1 tbs fresh butter

Whisk all ingredients (except for butter) together well; if necessary, beat the egg whites to snow and fold in last. Heat the butter in the omelette pan, add the egg mixture and stir lightly with a fork. When the mixture is semi-solid, push together on one side, finish baking and turn out onto a hot plate. The omelette should still be moist.

Omelette, French, with tomatoes
Ingredients and preparation according to recipe above.
1 tomato
½ tbs health food store vegetable fat
1 tbs chopped onion

Sauté the onion in the vegetable fat, add the peeled and diced tomato, and cook until the juice is reduced.
Cut into the omelette in the middle and pour on the finished tomatoes.

Shortcrust
200 g flour
80–100 g butter
1 tbs fruit sugar
1 egg

Spread the butter on the flour in fine flakes and grate finely. Add fructose and egg, knead lightly until a smooth dough is formed. Leave in a cool place for 30 minutes.

Sauces

Sauces are difficult for inclusion in a healing diet, since almost all recipes contain large amounts of fat (butter, oil, cream), cheese and eggs. The combination of hot fat and flour (béchamel sauce) should always be avoided, because this mixture is hard to digest. We have put together a few allowable sauces here whose recipes differ from the classic ones. All of them taste very good.

Béchamel sauce, classic (recipe 1)
1 tbs health food store vegetable fat
½ tbs butter
1 tbs flour
½ dl milk
½ dl vegetable broth or water
Pinch of sea salt (optional), nutmeg
Freshly ground white pepper

Heat butter and vegetable fat, sift in the flour and sauté lightly. Slowly add milk and vegetable broth while stirring constantly. Cook for 20 minutes. Salt and season.

Béchamel sauce with egg (recipe 2)
For 4 persons:
2–3 tbs wheat flour
1 l milk
1 bay leaf
1 tbs vegetable broth
1 grated onion
Pinch each of nutmeg and freshly ground white pepper
Chopped parsley

Briefly warm the flour without fat (it must not turn dark) until it gives off an appetising aroma, then let cool slightly. Add the milk, bay leaf, vegetable broth and onion while stirring constantly. Bring to a boil. Season to taste. After approx. 5 minutes, remove the bay leaf and serve the sauce sprinkled with parsley.

This basic sauce can be used to make many different versions. For example:

Béchamel sauce (recipe 3)
For 4 persons:
2 tbs wheat flour
½ l soy milk
1 bay leaf
1 onion, finely grated
2 tsp red miso
Pinch each of pepper and paprika
Chopped parsley

Briefly brown the flour without fat until it gives off a toasty aroma. Leave to cool briefly then add the soy milk while stirring constantly. Add the bay leaf and onion, and boil for about 5 minutes. Stir in the miso, remove the bay leaf and season the sauce with pepper and paprika. Sprinkle with chopped parsley.
(Miso is a fermented soybean paste that is excellent for seasoning. It tastes like soy sauce but does not contain salt.)

Horseradish sauce
To finish with, add 10 g finely grated horseradish and cook the sauce for another 5 minutes.

Caper sauce
Season the finished sauce with whole or chopped capers and lemon juice.

Olive sauce
Briefly cook the sauce with 4–5 tbs tomato pulp and 2 tbs chopped olives. Season with a pinch of cayenne pepper (optional).

Herb sauce
Mix a large amount of finely chopped herbs (e.g. parsley, lovage, chervil, basil, estragon, oregano) into the finished sauce.

Mushroom sauce
Mix 3–4 tbs of very finely chopped raw mushrooms into the finished sauce and season with lemon juice.

Tomato sauce, classic recipe
½ tbs health food store vegetable fat
1 tbs onion
½ garlic clove, pressed
2 tbs carrots, celery root (celeriac)*, leek
2 small tomatoes
Pinch of whole cane sugar (or Succanat)
1 tsp tomato puree

1 ½ dl vegetable broth or water
Bay leaf, rosemary, thyme

Sauté the chopped onion, pressed garlic and coarsely cut vegetables in vegetable fat. Add the diced tomatoes and the tomato puree. Then add vegetable broth or water, season and simmer for 30 minutes. Strain if desired.

* Omit if on a strict sodium-free diet.

Tomato sauce, simple
3 tomatoes
Small amount of miso
Pinch of whole cane sugar (or Succanat)
Chives, basil
1 tbs olive oil

Dice tomatoes, sauté until soft, season and drain. Add olive oil to taste.

Onion sauce
½ health food store margarine
1 small onion
1 tbs flour
1 dl vegetable broth
Small amount of nut spread
Nutmeg, miso or Kelpamare

Sauté the onions cut in strips in the margarine, sprinkle flour over the onions and cover with vegetable broth. Cook for 20 minutes. Season to taste. Strain the finished sauce if desired and add nut spread to refine.

Brown sauce
½ tbs health food store vegetable fat
1 tbs flour
1 dl vegetable broth
Clove powder, lemon juice, nutmeg

Roast the flour until it is chestnut brown, let cool. Add vegetable broth and cook for 20 minutes. Season to taste.

Mayonnaise, classic recipe
For 4 persons:
1 egg yolk
1 tbs lemon juice
2 dl oil
Onion, herbs and a small amount of Kelpamare

Mix the egg yolk well with several drops of lemon juice. Add the oil drop by drop while whisking evenly. If the mayonnaise becomes too thick, dilute with lemon juice. Season to taste.

Mayonnaise without animal protein
See recipe page 60.

Remoulade sauce, classic recipe
For 4 persons:
Prepare mayonnaise according to above recipe.
1 hard-boiled egg, chopped
1 tbs cornichons, chopped
Small amount of capers
1 tsp parsley, chopped
Tomato, diced

Mix the various ingredients with the finished mayonnaise. Garnish with diced tomato.

Remoulade sauce without animal protein
For 4 persons:
Prepare mayonnaise without animal protein and fat (see recipe page 60) and mix with 1 tbs chopped cornichons, capers and chopped parsley. Garnish with diced tomato.

Vinaigrette
For 4 persons:
2 tbs olive oil
2 tbs ground nut oil
2 ½ tbs lemon juice
2 dl water or vegetable broth
½ onion, chopped
1 egg, hard-boiled and chopped
1–2 cornichons, cut or finely chopped

Parsley or chives
1 tbs tomato, diced

Whisk oil, lemon juice and vegetable broth until smooth, then add the other ingredients while mixing thoroughly.

Sandwiches

Sandwiches are popular as appetisers, for a summer meal, to take along on hikes and journeys, and as lunch at the office. Spreads and ingredients can be used in any number of ways, and various wholemeal types of bread are available, some pre-sliced. Salt-free toast should be at least one day old before you slice it thinly.
The recipes are for 4 persons.

Basic spreads
For the strict diet, simply spread some quark on the bread rolls and add raw food.

Guacamole (avocado mousse)*
2 ripe avocados
Juice of ½ lemon
½ small onion, chopped
2 garlic cloves, pressed
Small amount of rock salt and white pepper (optional)

Mash the flesh removed from the avocados together with the lemon juice in a blender. Add the onion and garlic, and season with rock salt and white pepper. If desired, stir in 1 tbs soy cream (instead of crème fraîche).

* Omit if on a strict sodium-free diet.

Sweet avocado cream
1 ripe avocado
4 tbs fresh orange juice
1 tbs honey
Pinch of ginger powder

Mash the pulp removed from the avocado by squeezing it out or blending it, and mix in the other ingredients. Serve at once.

Tofu spread with nuts
250 g tofu, pureed
2 finely chopped spring onions
50 g nuts (hazelnuts, walnuts, almonds, cashew nuts)
Sea salt and white pepper (optional)

Lightly roast the nuts in the oven or an ungreased pan, let cool. Grind the roasted nuts and mix with the pureed tofu and onion. Season with sea salt and pepper.

Quark spread with herbs
100 g quark
10 g health food store vegetable margarine
Kelpamare or miso
Caraway, chives or herbs (dill, borage, lovage,
basil, oregano, peppermint, etc.)

Beat quark and vegetable margarine to a frothy consistency, season and add individual herbs (or a mix).

Garnishes
Spreads can be garnished with raw carrots or celery root (celeriac)* with tomatoes, fresh cucumbers, radish, cress, onion rings, nuts, parsley, chives, etc.

* Omit if on a strict sodium-free diet.

Mushroom toasts
2 pieces of salt-free toast bread
½ tbs health food store vegetable fat

1 tomato
1 egg, hard-boiled
Mushroom sauce

Bake toast in vegetable fat until golden brown. Cut tomato into thick slices, stew briefly. Place 2 slices of tomato on each of the slices, topped with a few slices of egg and pour over the mushroom sauce (see recipe on page 59).

Open-faced cheese sandwich
2 wholemeal bread slices, salt-free
½ dl milk
½ tbs health food store vegetable fat
1 tbs flour
1 dl milk
50 g salt-free cheese, grated
½ egg

Turn the bread slices in flour and place them on a greased baking tray. Prepare a béchamel sauce (recipe pages 59) with vegetable fat, flour and milk. Mix the cheese with the cooled sauce and spread on the bread slices. Bake in a hot oven for about 10 minutes.

Desserts
The following recipes are for 4 persons.

Desserts should be eaten with great restraint. Use honey (acacia honey is especially good), maple syrup, agave juice, fruit sugar or whole cane sugar (Succanat, Panela, etc.), though the latter is not suitable for all sweet dishes because of its strong taste. Do not eat any sweet dishes with large quantities of sugar, eggs or cream. There are many tasty alternatives.

Fruit salad
2 tbs honey
1 dl water
1–2 dl grape juice or apple juice
1–2 tbs lemon juice
600 g apricots or peaches
Melons
Apples
Pears (ripe)
Red cherries, pitted
Berries

Heat water with honey, grape juice and lemon juice and let cool. Thinly slice seasonal fruits and add them to the syrup.

Filled melons
2 small melons
Fruit salad as above

Halve the melons, scoop out the seeds and fill the melons with the fruit salad.

Fruit jelly
3 dl water or grape juice
1–2 tbs honey
10 g agar-agar, powdered
7 dl orange or berry juice

Mix water, honey and agar-agar, and cook over low heat while stirring constantly until the agar-agar has dissolved. Add fruit juice and serve immediately in glasses or desert bowls. Garnish with sesame cream to taste (see recipe page 38).

Agar-agar is a plant-based gelatine powder used for vegetable and fruit spreads, sauces, puddings, etc. as an alternative to animal gelatine.

Apple puree
800 g apples
2 dl water or apple juice
1–2 tbs honey
Cinnamon or lemon zest
1 dl sesame cream (see recipe page 38)

Remove stems and calyx from the apples, cut the apples into pieces, cook in water or apple juice until soft, and strain. Mix with cinnamon or lemon zest (from untreated lemons). To enrich, serve sesame cream with the apple puree.

Apple or pear compote
800 g apples or pears
2–3 dl water or apple juice
1 tbs honey
Grated lemon zest (untreated lemon) or cinnamon

Core and peel the apples or pears, and cut them into wedges. Bring water or apple juice to a boil, add honey and lemon zest or cinnamon, add apples or pears, and cook until soft.

Baked apples (1st recipe)
800 g apples
½ l water or apple juice
1 tbs honey
¼ cinnamon stick
Quince, raspberry or
currant jelly
or raisins and wine berries with a touch of honey

Boil water or apple juice with honey and cinnamon stick. Peel, halve and core apples, add them to the hot juice in portions. Cook slowly until soft. Remove with skimmer and place on a flat platter with the cut surface upwards. Fill the apples with jelly or mix of raisin, wine, berry and honey.

Baked apples (2nd recipe)
4 large or 8 small apples
4 tbs hazelnuts, ground
2 tbs currants
4 tbs sesame cream (see recipe page 38)
1–2 tbs honey
Grated lemon zest (untreated lemon)
10 g butter, vegetable margarine or nut spread
1 tbs whole cane sugar
1–2 dl apple juice

Mix hazelnuts, currants, sesame cream, honey and lemon zest, fill the prepared apples (cored, peeled and scored) and place the apples in a casserole. Add butter, vegetable margarine (or nut spread) and sugar, and pour 1 cm apple juice over the apples. Bake for 20–30 minutes.

Dried fruit salad with grapes and pine nuts
200 g dried figs
200 g dates
200 g dried apples
400 g white grapes
Juice of 1 lemon
2 tbs honey
50 g pine nuts

Chop the dried fruit, halve one-half of the grapes and squeeze the others. Place all fruits in a dish. Thoroughly mix the lemon juice and grape juice with the honey, and pour over the fruits. Cool before serving. Toast the pine nuts and sprinkle over the fruit salad.

Strawberry coupe
500 g strawberries
80–80 g fruit sugar
1–2 dl cream

Mix the berries or strain them through a very fine sieve. Add the fructose and mix thoroughly with the whipped cream. Garnish with whole berries.
Other fruits can also be used in this way.

Fruit coupe
250 g fruit (pears, apricots, peaches and berries)
2 dl water
2 tbs fruit sugar
½ portion vanilla cream
1 dl cream

Cook a compote with the fruit, water, and fructose. Pour the vanilla cream (see recipe page 64) on the fruit and garnish with whipped cream.

Heitisturm (blueberry mash)
Slightly constipating.
1 kg blueberries
80–100 g fruit sugar
2 dl water
1 tbs flour
2 tsp water
30 g butter
20 g bread cubes

Wash the blueberries and cook them with water and fruit sugar for 5–10 minutes. Stir the flour into the water, add to the cooked blueberries, cook and prepare. Toast the bread cubes lightly in butter and add to the blueberries.

Strawberry or raspberry cream
300 g berries
Vanilla cream
1–2 dl cream or sesame cream (see recipe page 38)

Prepare a vanilla cream according to the recipe on page 64 and add to the mixed or pureed berries. Add cream or sesame cream or serve separately.

Rhubarb crème
400 g rhubarb
80–100 g fruit sugar
Vanilla cream (see recipe page 64)

Wash the rhubarb, cut into cubes and cook until soft. Blend or strain the rhubarb, and mix with the vanilla cream.

Lemon cream
¾ l milk
1–2 lemon(s), untreated
1 tbs cornflour or arrowroot flour
3 tbs milk
2 tbs honey
Cream or sesame cream (see recipe page 38) to taste

Slice lemon peel thinly and boil in milk. Add cornflour or arrowroot flour stirred with a small amount of cold milk, and boil briefly. Add honey and return to pan, stirring constantly, and heat almost to boil. Strain the cooled cream and add a few spoons of lemon juice and sesame cream to taste.

Orange cream
Prepare like lemon cream (see recipe above).

Orange cream (cold stirred)
Zest of one orange (of organic untreated fruit)
1 dl water
1 small tsp agar-agar powder
2 dl orange juice
1 tsp lemon juice
5 tbs fruit sugar
2 eggs
1–2 dl cream

Slowly heat water with orange skin and agar-agar until the agar-agar is completely dissolved. Mix with orange and lemon juice. Stir eggs with fruit sugar until smooth and mix with fruit cream. Beat the cream until stiff and fold in thoroughly. Prepare in coupes or glasses, and let stand for 1 hour.

Lemon cream (cold stirred)
Zest of one lemon (of organic untreated fruit)
1½ dl water
1 small tsp agar-agar powder
3–4 tbs lemon juice
5 tbs fruit sugar
2 eggs
1–2 dl cream

Prepare like orange cream.

Orange aspic
5 dl orange juice
5 g agar-agar, powdered (plant jelly instead of gelatine)
1 tbs fruit sugar

Thoroughly whisk 3 dl orange juice, agar-agar and sugar, and heat over a low flame while stirring constantly (do not boil) until the agar-agar has dissolved completely. Add the remaining orange juice and pour into chilled moulds. Let cool.

Vanilla cream, classic
¾ l milk
1 vanilla pod
1 tbs cornflour
3 tbs milk
3 eggs
40–80 g fruit sugar or honey

Boil the milk with the vanilla pod. Mix the cornflour with the milk and add to the boiling milk, boil briefly. Whisk the eggs and fructose, add a little boiling milk, pour back into the pan while whisking, then bring to a near boil.

Vanilla cream without egg
1 vanilla pod
¼ l water
40 g wheat flour
3 tbs honey
Approx. 200 ml soy milk

Cut into the vanilla pod with a sharp knife, scrape out the pulp and place it in the water to boil. Put the wheat flour in the vanilla water while stirring constantly, and let swell to a thick mash. Let cool slightly, then stir in the honey and soy milk. Depending on the amount of soy milk, you will get vanilla cream or vanilla sauce. Keep cool until serving.

Vanilla sauce
See vanilla cream (recipe above).

Apple cream
¼ l milk
½ vanilla pod
1 tbs cornflour
1 tbs milk
1 egg
1 tbs fruit sugar
400 g apples
½ l water or apple juice
2 tbs fruit sugar
Grated lemon zest (of untreated fruit)
1–2 dl cream

Prepare a vanilla cream from milk, vanilla pod, cornflour, egg and fructose on the basis of the above recipe. Cook apples with water or sweet cider, fructose and lemon zest to a thick apple sauce and mix with the vanilla cream. Whip the cream until stiff and fold in or garnish the cream with it.

Almond milk sauce
4 dl milk
50 g almonds or almond puree
2 tbs honey
1 tbs cornflour or arrowroot flour
2 tsp water

Boil milk with the peeled ground almonds (or almond puree) and honey. Stir cornflour or arrowroot flour in cold water and stir into the boiling milk. Mix the finished sauce.

Rose hip sauce
70 g rose hip puree
or rose hip pulp (available in health food stores)
2 dl water or grape juice
1–2 tbs honey
A few drops of lemon juice (optional)

Boil the ingredients together then add the lemon juice.

Red wine sauce (non-alcoholic)
2 dl water
Lemon or orange zest (untreated fruits)
1 cinnamon stalk
1 clove
1–2 tbs honey
2 dl red grape juice
20 g almonds

Boil water, peel, spices and honey together for a few minutes, then pass through a sieve. Add grape juice and heat (do not boil). Add peeled and sliced almonds.

Red fruit jelly (chilled soup)
7 dl currant, raspberry or strawberry juice
Strawberry juice
3 dl red grape juice or water
70 g semolina
1 tbs cornflour

Boil berry juice and grape juice together, stir in semolina and cornflour, and boil for ten minutes. Pour into a freshly rinsed pudding bowl and store in a cool place.

Serve with vanilla sauce (see recipe page 64) or almond milk sauce (see recipe page 65).

Red fruit jelly, Danish style
1 kg berries (raspberries, currants, strawberries or
pitted cherries, or mix)
1 l fruit juice (e.g. elderberry)
2 packs of agar-agar
Honey, to taste
½ tsp natural vanilla
Sesame cream, liquid (see recipe page 38)

Put cleaned and chopped (optional) fruits into a dish, mix with honey and vanilla. Heat the fruit juice with agar-agar as per instructions and pour the liquid over the fruits. Leave the fruit jelly to harden. Serve with sesame cream.

Apple fritters
4 tbs flour
5 tbs water
2 tbs apple juice
1 egg white
6 apples (Boskop)
Health food store vegetable fat
Fruit sugar and cinnamon

Make a smooth batter from flour, water and apple juice. Fold in the whisked egg white. Peel and core the apples and cut into slices of 1 cm. Deep fry in hot vegetable fat until light brown. Roll the finished fritters in the mixture of fruit sugar and cinnamon.

Semolina pudding
150 g semolina
½ dl milk
Pinch of salt
2 tbs fruit sugar
Grated lemon zest (of untreated fruit)
1 egg, beaten
40 g almonds, peeled and ground
30 g raisins
Raspberry sirup

Cook semolina porridge with semolina, milk, salt, and lemon zest; add the fructose last. Mix the beaten egg with the almonds and raisins into the semolina and pour into a pudding mould. Cool. Serve with raspberry syrup.

Lemon cobbler
80 g butter
125 g flour
4 dl milk
150 g fruit sugar
3 eggs
Grated lemon zest (of untreated fruit)
2 tbs lemon juice

Sauté the flour in the butter, add the milk and cook into a thick porridge. Mix in the remaining ingredients and pour into a buttered baking dish. First cook in a water bath for 20 minutes, then finish baking in the oven (approx. 20 minutes).

Curd cheese cobbler
40 g butter
4 tbs flour
3 dl milk, hot
500 g quark
2 eggs
80–50 g fruit sugar
40 g raisins
Grated lemon zest (of untreated fruit)
4 tbs cream

Sauté the flour in the butter, carefully add the hot milk, and cook for a few minutes. Add the curd cheese with the beaten eggs and the remaining ingredients to the flour-milk mixture. Pour into a baking dish and bake in the oven for 30–40 minutes.

Rice-lemon pudding
9 dl water
Juice of one lemon
Lemon peel, diced (from untreated fruit)
Pinch of salt
150 g fruit sugar (or Succanat)
150 g rice
2 dl cream

Boil water, lemon juice, and lemon. Add sugar and rice and boil for 30 minutes. Fold in the whipped cream and pour it into a cold-rinsed custard dish. Let cool.

Sesame bars
100 g Syramena sugar
2 tbs honey
100 g sesame seeds, whole (not ground)

Heat the sugar in a dry pan and stir until a light caramel forms. Add the liquid honey and mix well. Add the sesame and mix well. Pour into a mould or onto an oiled board, let cool slightly, and cut into squares or diamonds. Let cool.

Syramena sugar is a light-coloured raw cane sugar available in health food stores.

Oatmeal biscuits
200 g oat flakes
100 g butter
1 egg
200 g fruit sugar (or Succanat)
Vanilla sugar
100 g flour

Roast the oatmeal. Stir butter and egg until frothy. Mix with the rolled oats and the remaining ingredients to form a soft dough. Roll the dough out to a thickness of 3 mm, cut out, brush with egg yolk and bake over a medium heat.

Swabian rolls
150 g butter
200 g Succanat or Syramena
100 g hazelnuts, roasted and ground
350 g wholemeal flour
1–2 eggs
Juice and zest of one lemon (from untreated fruit)
Pinch of cinnamon
Pinch of salt

Stir butter and sugar until frothy. Mix with the remaining ingredients to form a soft dough and leave in a cool place for 1 hour. Cut out as desired, brush with egg yolk and bake on medium heat.

Healthy Teas

Use whole leaves for teas if possible, since the essential oils are lost when leaves are finely chopped (as in a tea bag). Bitter and flatulence teas are drunk unsweetened; other teas can have honey and/or diluted lemon juice added.

Bitter tea
Wormwood
Centaurium (goldenrod)
Blessed thistle
Mix in equal parts, boil briefly and steep for 5 minutes.
To stimulate the appetite, drink 2–3 tbs 30 minutes before meals.
Mildly cholagogue, aids in digestion.
Sensitive persons should use only centaurium (goldenrod, prepared like camomile tea).

Wormwood tea
Add hot water and steep for 5 minutes.
Strong bitter tea, highly cholagogue, stimulates gastric juices.
Sip throughout the day.

Flatulence tea
Caraway (optional)
Fennel
Aniseed
Mix in equal parts, add hot water and steep for 20 minutes.
Drink 1 cup after meals to prevent flatulence.

Chamomile tea
Steep very briefly.
Drink for stomach pain.
Cleansing and calming effect on the gastrointestinal tract.
For enemas and rinsing.

Peppermint tea
Steep briefly.
Calming, cholagogue, stimulating effect on small intestine.

Vervain tea
Steep briefly.
Calming, mucous reducing, cholagogue.
In the afternoon and evening.
Very popular in France.

Solidago tea (goldenrod, pagan woundwort)
Boil for 1 minute, steep for 10 minutes.
For dropsy, bladder and kidney infections. Water expelling. Drink 2–3 cups per day.

Bearberry leaf tea
Simmer 1 ½ tbs bearberry leaf tea in 5 dl water for 5 minutes, steep for 10 minutes, strain. For bladder infections.

Bergamot tea
Steep briefly.
Very calming, good before bedtime as well.

Orange blossom tea
Boil 2–3 blossoms for 2–3 minutes, let steep and strain. Sweeten with honey.
Calming. Drink before bedtime.

Lemon peel tea
For 2 cups peel 1 organic untreated lemon into thin strips. Add boiling water, let steep for 5 minutes then strain. Drink with a small amount of honey before going to bed.

Flaxseed tea
Boil 1 tbs flaxseed in ½ l water for 7–10 minutes and let steep briefly.
Mucous reducing, mildly laxative, stomach soothing.

Lavender tea
Add hot water 1 tsp lavender leaves, steep briefly.
Calming, harmonising, anti-inflammatory, for insomnia.

Rose hip tea
Soak 2–3 tbs of rose hip seeds and shells in 1 ½ l water for 12 hours, simmer for 30–45 minutes then strain. The remaining rose hips can be reused with fresh ones the next day.
Slightly cholagogue and diuretic, refreshing, stimulating.

Blueberry tea
Soak 1 tbs of dried blueberries for 12 hours and boil for 5 minutes. Strain.
Astringent, calming.

Table Regarding Glycaemic Index and Glycaemic Charge

The glycaemic index indicates how quickly and how high the blood glucose level will climb when a certain food is eaten. It is expressed in the percentage of the rise caused by the same amount of glucose.

The glycaemic charge is calculated by taking the glycaemic index and multiplying it by the content of pure carbohydrates. If a food has a high glycaemic index and consists mainly of pure carbohydrates, it has a very high glycaemic charge. If it mostly contains pure carbohydrates that are converted into glucose, the food will need a large quantity of insulin to enter the cells and let the blood sugar level settle again.

Only those carbohydrates that are converted into glucose, and therefore need insulin to be absorbed into cells, will produce a blood glucose increase after a meal. Other sugar types, such as those in fruits and vegetables which are not converted into glucose (fructose, sorbitol, etc.), do not increase the glycaemic index and do not require insulin. The glycaemic index therefore provides the best information for calculating the insulin required to ingest a particular food for diabetics.

Because of the multiplication of the glycaemic index with the content of all pure carbohydrates, the glycaemic charge load contains all pure carbohydrates, including those that do not need insulin to be processed. Therefore it is less suitable for calculating insulin requirements than the glycaemic index. On the other hand, it has proved useful to take this into account, as it has been shown that foods with a high glycaemic charge also contribute to the glycation (glycation) of the inner layer of the blood vessels and have an unfavourable effect on the fat metabolism disorder by increasing the triglyceride level.

For prevention of arteriosclerosis and diabetes, ideally one should use foods that have a low glycaemic index and charge, and which are good food integrals. This is because their carbohydrate content should comprise mainly fructose and sugar types other than glucose, and whose glucose content can only be broken down slowly during digestion. These unheated fruits, vegetables, whole grains and nuts are part of a raw food regime.

Foods	Glycaemic index in %	Glycaemic charge
Amaranth	30	<10
Apple	38	5
Apple, dried	29	16
Apple juice, clear, bottled	40	5
Apple juice, naturally clouded	37	4
Apricots, dried	31	14
Apricots, fresh	57	4
Artichokes	20	2
Asparagus	20	<10
Aubergines	10	<10
Avocado	20	<10
Baguette, white bread	70	36
Bananas	52	10
Barley	43	12
Basmati rice	58	15
Beans, black	42	8
Beans, cooked white	48	5
Beans (kidney)	28	5
Beetroot (red beet), cooked	64	47
Bran bread	50	10
Broccoli	10	<10
Buckwheat	54	11
Bulgur, cooked	48	8
Buttermilk natural <10	<10	<10
Cabbage	10	0
Carrots, cooked	85	3
Carrot juice, bottled	43	4
Carrots, raw	47	4
Celery tubers, cooked	43	24
Cherries	22	2

Foods	Glycaemic index in %	Glycaemic charge
Chick peas, cooked	38	6
Chocolate whole milk	15	0
Corn flour (polenta)	69	6
Corn, popcorn	72	40
Corn (sweet corn)	54	11
Cornflakes	81	70
Courgette	15	<10
Couscous	65	15
Crackers	67	38
Dried dates	103	69
Figs, fresh	40	?
Figs, dried	61	21
Fruit (average value)	35–45	3–10
Fruit bread	47	24
Fruit yoghurt, sugared	40	6
Fruit yoghurt, sweetener	14	1
Garlic	10	<10
Gluten-free light bread	76	38
Grapefruit	25	2
Grapefruit juice, bottled	48	4
Green beans (mung beans)	38	?
Green salads	10	0
Green spelt	55	?
Hamburger bun	85	31
Honey	55	40
Horseradish	35	<10
Ice cream, full cream	61	13
Jam (marmalade)	51	34

Foods	Glycaemic index in %	Glycaemic charge
Jasmine scented rice	109	31
Kiwi	50	5
Kohlrabi, cooked	70	5
Lean quark	10	1
Leek	10	<10
Lemons	70	33
Lentils, green cooked	30	3
Lentils, red cooked	26	3
Long-grain rice	56	16
Mango	51	7
Mars bar	65	43
Melon (honeydew melon)	65	3
Milk bread roll ("Weggli")	63	34
Milk, partially skimmed	32	2
Milk, whole	27	1
Millet, cooked	71	17
Muesli flakes, industrial	49	33
Muffin	53	30
Mushrooms	15	0
Natural yoghurt	35	1–5
Nectarine	30	<10
Nutella	33	20
Nuts (average)	25	1–5
Nuts, cashew	22	3
Nuts, peanuts	15	2
Oat bran	55	28
Oat bran bread	47	28
Oat flakes	59	36
Oatmeal bread	65	41
Oat porridge	60	8
Onions	10	<10

Foods	Glycaemic index in %	Glycaemic charge
Oranges	42	4
Orange juice, bottled	50	5
Papaya	59	8
Parboiled rice	47	11
Parsnip	10	<10
Pasta (average)	56	42
Pasta egg noodles	33	8
Pasta rice noodles	40	10
Pasta soy glass noodles	60	40
Pasta spaghetti (al dente)	61	13
Pasta spaghetti (soft)	44	12
Pasta whole-wheat (al dente)	61	15
Peach	42	4
Pears	38	9
Peas (fresh)	40	4
Persimmon	50	8
Pineapples	59	6
Pineapple juice, bottled	46	6
Plums	39	4
Plums, dried	29	16
Potatoes, baked	85	17
Potatoes, boiled	78	11
Potatoes, crisps	54	23
Potatoes, French fries	75	15
Potatoes, gnocchi	68	18
Potatoes in their skins (boiled)	85	3
Potatoe mash	74	10
Potatoe mash from powder	85	11

Foods	Glycaemic index in %	Glycaemic charge
Potatoes, new	57	8
Potatoes, sweet potatoes	61	11
Pretzel	83	48
Pumpernickel	50	20
Pumpkin, cooked	75	4
Quinoa	35	?
Radish	35	1
Radishes	30	<10
Raisins	58	27
Raisins	15	0
Rice Krispies (Kellogg)	82	71
Rice Krispies	82	71
Risotto rice	69	24
Rutabaga, yellow	70	7
Rye crispbread	64	41
Rye sourdough bread	50	30
Rye wholemeal bread	53	21
Sauerkraut	65	3
Semolina	65	4

Foods	Glycaemic index in %	Glycaemic charge
Shortbread biscuit	51	37
Soybean, cooked	85	2
Soybean sprouts	18	1
Sponge cake	46	26
Strawberries	40	1
Sweet peppers	65	10
Vegetable juice, bottled	43	2
Wheat semolina (white)	37	9
Wheat sprouts	60	7
Wheat coarse meal	60	9
Whey, natural	<10	<10
White rice	64	15
White wheat bread	75	50
Wholemeal rye bread	35	26
Wholemeal rye bread	10	<10
Yoghurt drink	38	6
Yoghurt, natural	36	2

List of Recipes

Almond milk	37
– from fresh almonds	37
Almond milk sauce	65
Almond puree	38
Almond puree dressing	34
Apple cream	65
Apple fritters	66
Apple muesli	30
Apple muesli with almond or sesame puree	31
Apple muesli with cream	31
Apple muesli with yoghurt, sour milk or buttermilk	30
Apple or pear compote	62
Apple puree	62
Apples (baked)	
– 1st recipe	63
– 2nd recipe	63
Artichokes	48
Asparagus	48
Aubergines (eggplant)	48
Avocado	
– guacamole	61
– sweet avocado cream	61
Baked fennel with cream cheese crème	44
Beans, green with tomatoes	45
Bearberry leaf tea	68
Béchamel sauce	
– classic recipe 1	59
– recipe 3	59
– with egg, recipe 2	59
Beetroot (red beet)	46
Bergamot tea	68
Bitter tea	67
Black salsify, sautéed	46
Blueberry tea	68
Broccoli	48
Brussels sprouts, sautéed	49
Butter	38
Butter dumplings	40
Cabbage or white cabbage, sautéed	49
Carrots and peas	45
Cauliflower	48
Celery root (celeriac)	
– sautéed	46
– with béchamel sauce	46
Celery root (celeriac)-apple-banana-raw food	35
Celery root (celeriac) salad with soy mayonnaise	51
Celery stalks	44
Chamomile tea	67
Chervil soup	42
Chestnut vegetables	50
Coarse-ground grain mash	57
Colewort	49
Cooked carrots	45
Cooked snow peas (sugar peas)	45
Cooked sugar peas (snow peas)	45
Cooking and steaming, gentle	39
Courgette and tomato medley	47
Cream dressing	33
Curd cheese cobbler	66
Desserts	62
Dressings and herbs to go with raw vegetables	36
Dried fruit salad with grapes and pine nuts	63
Endive/chicory	44
Flatulence tea	67
Flaxseed tea	68
Fruit coupe	63
Fruit jelly	62
Fruit salad	62
Grain Dishes	54
Gruel added to juices	30
Guacamole (avocado mousse)	61

Healthy Teas	67	Open-faced cheese sandwich	62
Heitisturm (blueberry mash)	63	Orange aspic	64
Herbal soup	40	Orange blossom tea	68
		Orange cream	64
Jerusalem artichoke	46	– cold stirred	64
Juices	29		
		Pancake strips	40
Knöpfli		Pasta, noodles, spaghetti, macaroni etc.	57
– without egg	57	Peas and carrots	45
– with spinach or tomato	57	Peas, French style	45
Kohlrabi with herbs	49	Peppermint tea	68
		Pine nut milk	37
Lavender tea	68	Polenta	56
Leek cream soup	42	Polenta slices	56
Leeks	50	Potato	
Lemon cobbler	66	– dumplings	53
Lemon cream	64	Potato cakes	53
– cold stirred	64	Potato chips	54
Lemon peel tea	68	Potato dishes	51
Lentils	50	Potatoes	
		– ayurvedic	54
Mayonnaise	34, 60	– baked	52
– classic recipe	34	– bouillon potatoes	52
– quark mayonnaise	34	– in their skins	51
– without animal protein	60	– Lyonnaise style	53
– with wholemeal soy flour		– princess potatoes	53
instead of egg	34	– puree	53
Melon, filled	62	– roasted	53
Milk types	37	– with caraway	52
Millet risotto	57	– with cream	52
– with vegetables	57	– with kale	54
Minestrone	43	– with quark	52
Muesli		– with tomatoes	52
– with berries and stone fruit	31	Potato goulash	54
– with condensed milk	31	Potato mash	52
– with dried fruits	31	Potato salad	50
– with various fruits	31	– with cucumbers	50
Mushroom toasts	61	Potato soup	43
Nut spread	38	Quark dressing, spicy	34
		Quark mayonnaise	34
Oat cream soup	41	Quark spread	
Oat flake dumplings	58	– with herbs	61
Oat groat soup	41	Quark-yoghurt dressing	33
Oil dressing	33		
Omelette	58	Ratatouille	48
– french	58	Raw vegetables	35
– french, with tomatoes	58	– mixed	35
Onion soup	42	– mixed and pureed	36

Raw vegetables and salads		– tomato sauce, classic recipe	59
– freshness and quality	32	– tomato sauce, simple	60
– harmonious composition	32	Sauerkraut salad	35
– thorough cleaning	32	Sautéed chicory/endive	44
Red beet (beetroot)	46	Semolina dumplings	40
Red cabbage	49	Semolina gnocchi	56
Red fruit jelly		Semolina mash	56
– chilled soup	65	Semolina pudding	66
– Danish style	66	Semolina soup	41
Red wine sauce (non-alcoholic)	65	Sesame bars	67
Remoulade sauce		Sesame cream	38
– classic recipe	60	Sesame frappé (shake)	38
– without animal protein	60	Sesame milk	37
Rhubarb crème	64	Sesame puree dressing	34
Rice		Shortcrust	58
– Indian rice dish	56	Solidago tea (goldenrod, pagan woundwort)	68
– Japanese	54		
– rice gratin with tomatoes	55	Soup additions	40
– rice-lemon pudding	66	Soups	39
– rice salad	51	Soy milk	38
– risotto	54	Spätzle (without egg)	57
– riz creole with vegetables	55	Spinach	
– with courgettes	55	– chopped	43
– with peas (risi e bisi)	55	– whole leaves	43
– with saffron	55	Sprouted cereal grains	35
– with spinach	55	Strawberry Coupe	63
– with tomatoes	55	Strawberry or raspberry cream	64
Rice soup		Swabian rolls	67
– clear	40	Sweet dishes	62
– thickened	40	Sweet peppers (green, yellow, red)	47
Romaine lettuce	43	Swiss chard	
Rose hip sauce	65	– or false asparagus	44
Rose hip tea	68	– with béchamel sauce	44
Salad dressings	33	Tofu spread with nuts	61
– sweet and sour	35	Tomatoes	
Salad dressings, to go with, table	36	– à la provençale	47
Salade niçoise	51	– baked	47
Salads of cooked vegetables	50	– raw, stuffed	35
Sandwiches	61	– stewed	46
– basic spreads	61	– stuffed	47
– garnishes	61	– with cheese slices	47
Sauces	58, 59	Tomato soup	41
– brown sauce	60	– summer	42
– caper sauce	59		
– horseradish sauce	59	Vanilla cream	
– mushroom sauce	59	– classic	64
– olive sauce	59	– without egg	65
– onion sauce	60	Vegetable aspic	51

Vegetable broth	39	Vegetable stock	39
Vegetable curry	45	Vervain tea	68
Vegetable fats, unhardened	38	Vinaigrette	60
Vegetables	43		
Vegetable soups	42	Wormwood tea	67
– carrots, spinach, broccoli, cauliflower	42	Yoghurt dressing	33

Notes

1. Stöllner T.: Salz, Salzgewinnung, Salzhandel. 3. Archäologisches. In: Reallexikon der Germanischen Altertumskunde. 2nd edition; volume 26, 2004: 357–79
2. Bass H.H.: *Hungerkrisen in Preussen während der ersten Hälfte des 19. Jahrhunderts.* Scripta Mercatureas, Verlag St. Katharinen 1991 ISBN 3-922661-90-4, 124
3. Borst J.G. et al.: *Hypertension explained by Starling's theory of circulatory homeostasis.* Lancet 1963; 1: 677–82
4. Guyton A.C. et al.: *Long-term regulation of the circulation: intervention ship with body fluid volumes.* In: Reeve E. et al.: Physical basis of circulatory transport: regulation and exchange. Philadelphia: Saunders; 1967. 137–201
5. Ambard L. et al.: *Causes de l'hypertension artérielle.* Arch Gen Med 1904; 1: 520–33
6. Kempner W.: *Treatment of hypertensive vascular disease with the rice diet.* Am. J. Med. 1948; 4: 545–77
7. Ball O.T. et al.: *Observations on dietary sodium chloride.* Am J Diet Assoc 1957; 33: 366–70
8. Dahl et al.: *Effects of chronic salt ingestion. Evidence that genetic factors play an important role in susceptibility to experimental hypertension.* J Exp Med 1962; 115: 1173–90
9. Denton B et al.: *The effect of increased salt intake on blood pressure of chimpanzees.* Nat Med 1995; 1: 1009–16
10. Mac Gregor G.A. et al.: *Double blind randomised crossover trial of moderate sodium restriction in essential hypertension.* Lancet 1982; 1: 351–55
11. Intersalt Cooperative Research Group: *Intersalt: an international study of electrolyte excretion and blood pressure. Results for 24 h urinary sodium and potassium excretion.* BMJ 1988; 297: 319–28
12. The Trials of Hypertension Prevention Collaborative Research Group: the effects of nonpharmacologic interventions on blood pressure and hypertension incidence in overweight people with high-normal blood pressure. JAMA 1992; 267: 1213–20
13. The Trials of Hypertension Prevention Collaborative Research Group: *Effects of weight loss and sodium reduction intervention on blood pressure and hypertension incidence in overweight people with high-normal blood pressure: the Trials of Hypertension Prevention phase II.* Arch Intern Med 1997; 157: 657–67
14. Whelton P.K. et al.: *For the TONE Collaborative Research Group. Sodium reduction and weight loss in the treatment of hypertension in older persons. A randomized controlled trial of nonpharmacologic interventions in the elderly (TONE).* JAMA 1998; 279: 837–46
15. Sacks F.M. et al.: *DASH-Sodium Collaborative Research Group: Effects on blood pressure of reduced dietary sodium and the dietary approaches to stop hypertension (DASH)-Diet.* N Engl J Med 2001; 344: 3–10
16. He J. et al.: *Dietary sodium intake and subsequent risk of cardiovascular disease in overweight adults.* JAMA 1999; 282: 2027–34
17. Tuomilehto J. et al.: *Urinary sodium excretion and cardiovascular mortality in Finland: a prospective study.* Lancet 2001; 357: 848–51
18. Cook N.R. et al.: *Long term effects of dietary sodium reduction on cardiovascular disease outcomes: observational follow up of the trials of hypertension prevention (TOHP).* BMJ 2007; 334: 885–88
19. Strazzullo P. et al.: *BMJ 2009; 339: b4567–b4376*
20. Kawasaki T. et al.: *The effect of high-sodium and low-sodium intakes on blood pressure and other related variables in human subjects with idiopathic hypertension.* Am J Med 1978; 64: 193–98
21. Luft F.C. et al.: *Cardiovascular and humoral responses to extremes of sodium intake in normal black and white men.* Circulation 1979; 60: 697–706
22. Weinberger M.H. et al.: *Definitions and characteristics of sodium sensitivity and blood pressure resistance.* Hypertension 1986; 8 (suppl 2): II127–II134

23 Reineck J.H. et al.: *Regulation of sodium balance.* In: Maxwell M.H. and Kleeman C.R. editors. Clinical disorders of fluid and electrolyte metabolism. New York, McGraw-Hill: 1980: 89–112

24 Weinberger M.H. et al.: *A comparison of two tests for the assessment of blood pressure responses to sodium.* Am J Hypertens 1993; 6: 179–84

25 Morimoto A. et al.: *Sodium sensitivity and cardiovascular events in patients with essential hypertension.* Lancet 1997; 350: 1734–37

26 Weinberger M.H. et al.: *Salt sensitivity, pulse pressure, and death in normal and hypertensive humans.* Hypertension 2001; 37: 429–32

27 He J. et al.: *Gender difference in blood pressure responses to dietary sodium intervention in the GenSalt study.* J Hypertens 2009; 27: 48–54

28 De Leeuw P.W. et al.: *Salt and sensitivity.* Hypertension 2013; 62: 461–62

29 Lifton R. et al.: *Molecular mechanisms of human hypertension.* Cell. 2001; 104: 545–56

30 Mu S. et al.: *Epigenetic modulations of the renal β-adrenergic-WNK-4 pathway in salt sensitive hypertension.* Nat Med 2011; 17: 573–80

31 Titze J. et al.: *Internal sodium balance in DOCA-salt rats: A body composition study.* Am J Physiol Renal Physiol 2005; 287: F793–F802

32 Titze J. et al.: *Glycose minoglycan polymerization may enable osmotically inactive Na+ storage in the skin.* Am J Physiol Heart Circ Physiol. 2004; 287: H203–H208

33 Machnik A. et al.: *Macrophages regulate salt dependent volume and blood pressure by a vascular endothelial growth factor-C-dependant buffering mechanism.* Nat Med 2009; 15: 545–52

34 Machnik A. et al.: *Mononuclear phagocyte system depletion blocks interstitial tonicity-responsive enhancer binding protein/vascular endothelial growth factor C expression and induces salt-sensitive hypertension in rats.* Hypertension 2010; 55: 755–76

35 Chappell D. et al.: *The Glycocalyx of the human umbilical vein endothelial cell: An impressive structure ex vivo but not in culture.* Circ Res 2009; 104: 1313–17

36 Oberleitner H. et al.: *Salt overload damages the glycocalyx sodium barrier of vascular endothelium.* Pflugers Arch 2011; 462–519:528

37 Oberleitner H. et al.: *Plasma sodium stiffens vascular endothelium and reduces nitric oxyde release.* Proc Natl Acad Sci U S A 2007; 104: 16281–86

38 Korte S. et al.: *Feedforward activation of endothelial ENaC by high sodium.* FASEB J 2014; 28: 4015–25

39 Lang F.: *Stiff endothelial cell syndrome in vascular inflammation and mineralocorticoid excess.* Hypertension 2011; 57: 146–47

40 Marx N.: *Pathophysiologie der Arteriosklerose bei Diabetes mellitus.* Clinical R 4 research in Cardiology Supplements, 1. 2006

41 Bircher-Benner M.O.: *Eine neue Ernährungslehre.* Wendepunkt Verlag Berlin, Leipzig, Zürich, 10th edition, 1945

42 Bircher-Benner M.O.: *Grundzüge der Ernährungstherapie auf Grund der Energie-Spannung der Nahrung.* Verlag Otto Salle, Berlin, 1905 and 1905.

43 Kasnacev V.P.: in Jezowska-Trzebiatovska B. et al.: Photon emission from biological systems, proceedings of the first international Symposium, Wroclav, Pland Jan. 1986

44 Bischof M.: *Biophotonen, das Licht in unseren Zellen.* ISBN 3-86150-095-7

45 Popp F.A.: *Biologie des Lichtes, Grundlagen der ultraschwachen Zellstrahlung.* Verlag Paul Parey, ISBN 3-489-61734-7

46 Popp F.A.: *Unsere Lebensmittel in neuer Sicht.* ISBN 3-596-11459-4

47 Van Vijck R. and E. Utrecht Univeriy: *An Introduction to Human Biophoton Emission.* Forsch Komplementärmed. Klass. Naturheilkd. 1005, 12, 77–83

48 Prigogine I. et al.: *Dialog mit der Natur.* Piper Verlag München, ISBN 3-492-11181-5

49 Pischinger A.: *Das System der Grundregulation, Grundlagen für eine ganzheitsbiologische Theorie der Mediin.* Huat-Verlag, Heidelberg, 1990. 8th expanded edition, ISBN 3-7760-1183-1

50 Jezowska-Trzebiatowska et al. *Photon emission from biological systems, proceedings of the first international Symposium,* Wroclav, Pland Jan, in Popp. F.A.: *Biologie des Lichtes, Grundlagen der ultraschwachen Zellstrahlung,* Paul Parey-Verlag, ISBN 3-489-61734-7

51 Bischof M.: *Biophotonen: das Licht in unseren Zellen.* Verlag 2001, ISBN 3-86150-095-7

52 Van Vijck R. et al.: *An Introduction to Human Biophoton Emission.* Utrecht University Forsch. klass. Naturheilkunde. 1005, 12, 77–83

53 Pischinger A.: *Das System der Grundregulation, Grundlagen für eine ganzheitsbiologische Theorie*

der Medizin, Haug-Verlag Heidelberg, 1990, ISBN 3-7760-1183-1

54 Bircher-Benner M.O.: *Die Verhütung des Unheilbaren.* Wendepunkt-Verlag Zürich, Leipzig, Wien, 2nd edition, 58

55 Kollenbach D.: Maximilian Oskar Bircher-Benner (1867–1939), Dissertation, Verlag der Medizinischen Fakultät der Universität Köln, 1974

Index

β-amyloid plaques	15	Blood volume	10, 11
β-amyloids	21	Bromine radical (Br*)	15
		Butter, vegetable fats and oils	38
Aarthritis	21		
Acetylcholine	12	Calcium flow	15
Acupuncture	20	Calories	17, 18, 23
Adhesion of the monocytes	12	Cancer	14, 21
Adipokines	13	Carbohydrates	23, 69
Aging process, premature	14	Cardiovascular disease	11
Aldosterone	8	Catalase	14
Alzheimer's disease	21	Cataract	21
Alzheimer's disease (AD)	15	Causes, genetic	11
Amyloids	21	Cell death, programmed (apoptosis)	15
Amyotrophic lateral sclerosis (ALS)	15	Chaperons	15
Angiotensin	8	Chloride radical (Cl*)	15
Angiotensin converting enzyme (ACE)	8	Chlorophyll A-molecules	18
		Chlorophyll funnels	18
Angiotensin I	8	Cholesterol	10, 21
Angiotensin II	8	Circulation, enterohepatic	21
Antidiuretic hormone (ADH)	8	Civilisation diseases	20
Apparatus, juxtaglomerular	8	Cleaning leafy vegetables	32
Arterioles	8	Cleaning root vegetables	32
Arteriosclerosis	12, 21	Cleaning vegetable fruits	32
Autoimmune reactions	21	Coagulation of the blood	12
		Coenzyme Q 10	14
Bacteria, anaerobic	20	Coherence	18, 19
Balance, thermodynamic	19	Collagen	13
Basedow	21	Connective tissue, soft	19
Basedow's thyroiditis	21	Cooking and steaming, gentle	39
Basic regulation	20	Cravings for salt	8
Basic regulation system	19, 20	Cytochrome C	15
Beta folding sheet structure, insoluble	15	Cytochrome P 450-oxidase	14
Bircher muesli	30		
Blood capillaries	19	Degeneration	21
Blood glucose levels	12	Desoxyribonucleic acid DNA)	18
Blood pressure	24	Desserts	62
Blood Pressure Regulation in the Kidney	8	Diabetes mellitus	12
		Diabetes mellitus type 2	17
Blood pressure value, diastolic	10	Diacylglycerol	13
Blood sugar level	69	Differentiation	18
Blood sugar levels	14	Diseases, degenerative	15

Diseases of civilisation	22	Glutathione	14
DNA peroxidation	14	Glutathione reductase	14
Dream phases	25	Glycation	12, 69
Dressings to go with salads and raw vegetables	36	Glycocalyx	10
		Glycolipids	10
Dysfunction, endothelial	10, 12, 13	Glycoproteids	10
		Grain Dishes	54
Effect of a Low-Salt Diet	11	Growth	18
Endothelin-1 (ET-1)	13	Gruel added to juices	30
Endothelium	12, 13		
Energy, chaotic	18	Haemorrhoids	21
Energy, orderly	18	Hashimoto's thyroiditis	21
Energy potential	22, 23	Health issues, mental	23
Entropy	17	Heart attack	12, 21
Epidemiological studies	11	Homoeostasis	12
Epigenetic Inheritance of Salt Sensitivity	11	Hunger	23
		Huntington's disease	15
Extracellular space	10	Hydrogen superoxide (H_2O_2)	14
		Hydroxide radical (OH*)	14
Fat metabolism disorder	69	Hydroxyl radical (OH*)	15
Fats (lipids with polyunsaturated fatty acids)	23	Hyperglycaemia	12
		Hypertension	24
Fattening diet	24	Hypertension, fixed	10, 13
Fatty acids, unsaturated	21	Hypertension, Order Therapy for	18
Fatty liver	20	Hypertension, salt-sensitive	10, 11
Fatty streaks	21		
Fears	23	Ideal weight	23, 24
Fibrinolysis	12	Immune competence	20
Fibronectin	13	Inflammation readiness	13
Food economy	21, 23	Inflammatory mediators	12
Food Economy	20	Information, biological	20, 22
Food energy	18	Information transfers	19
Food Energy	17	Insulin	69
Food integrals	69	Insulin level	13
Foods, living	17	Insulin resistance	13, 23
Foods, photon-containing	19	Integral law of nutrition	22
Free radicals (reactive oxygen species, ROS)	13, 14, 21	Intercellular space	10
		Intercellular substance	19, 21
Fresh foods, plant-based	19	Interference fields	20
Fructose	69	Interstitial fluid	19
		Intestinal flora	20
Garnishes	61		
Gene defects	11	Juices	29
Genetic material	18		
Glaucoma	21	Ketonic acid	21
Glucosamine molecules	11	Kidney failure, diabetic	21
Glucose	69		
Glucose metabolism	14	Laminin	13
Glutamate	15	Laser threshold	18, 19

81

Law on preservation of energy by Hermann von Helmholz	17
Leptin resistance	23
Lewy bodies	15
Life energy	19
Life information	19
Lipid peroxidation	14, 15
List of Recipes	73
Lymphangiogenesis	10
Lymph nodes	20
Lymph vessels	20
Macrophages	10, 11
Macula densa	8
Macular degeneration	21
Matrix	19, 20
Membrane lipids	10
Menus for the Low-Salt Diet	26
Mesangial cells	8
Metabolic balance	24
Metabolic slags, degenerative	20
Migration	12
Milk types	37
Mitochondria	14
Molecular sieve	19
Moleculs, aromatic	18
Monocytes	10
Movement	23
Multiple sclerosis (MS)	15
Muscle tension (tone)	12
Myelin sheaths	15
Myocardial infarction	11
NADP-oxydase	13
Nephrosis	21
Neuropathy, diabetic	15
Nitric oxide (NO)	11
Nitric oxide (NO*)	14
Nitrogen monoxide (NO)	12
Nitrogen oxide radical (NO*)	15
NMDA receptor	15
Non-REM sleep phase	25
NO-synthetase	15
Obesity	11, 17
Oral vein system	20
Order of Life	25
Osteoarthritis	21
Osteoporosis	21
Overeating	23
Overweight	11, 13
Oxidation	21
Oxidative stress	13
Oxygen deficit	12
Oxygen species, reactive	14
Parkinson's disease	15
Peroxide dismutase	14
Peroxinitrite (ONOO-)	13
Peroxynitrite	15
Perpetuum mobile	17
Phospholipids	10
Photons	18
Photon Storage	18
Photosyntheis	22
Physical exercise	25
Physical Exercise	25
Pituitary gland	8
Plant substances (phytochemicals)	14, 22
Plasminogen activator 1 (PA-1) and ET-1	13
Polysaccharides	10
Posterior lobe of the pituitary gland	8
Potassium	11
Potato dishes	51
Primary urine	8
Principle of chaos	19
Principle, ordering	19
Protein	23
Protein kinase C (PK-C)	13
Protein peroxidation	14
Proteoglycans	19, 20
Radiation, electromagnetic	14
Radiation, ionising	14
Radiation, UV-A	14
Raw food	23
Raw vegetables and salads	32
Raw vegetables, mixed, pureed	36
Regeneration	18
Relationship conflicts	23
REM phase	25
Renin	8, 11
Renin-Angiotensin-Aldosterone System	8
Resonance	19
Resonance, ordering	19
Respiratory chain	14

ROS (reactive oxygen species)	13, 14, 15, 21	Thermodynamics, second law of	17, 19
Rot (putrefaction) toxins	20	Tonicity response element binding protein (TonEBP)	10
Salad dressings	33	Trauma, mental	25
Salads of cooked vegetables	50	Triglyceride level	69
Salinisation	12	Tumour necrosis factor α (TNF-α)	13
Salt barrier	12	Type 1 diabetes mellitus	21
Salt, Osmotic Storage of	10	Type-II diabetes mellitus	13
Salt Storage	10		
Sandwiches	61	Ubiquinone	14
Sauces	58	Urinary tubule	8
Selenium	14	UV light	18
Sense of taste	23		
Sleep before midnight	23	Varicose veins	21
Sleepwalking	25	Vas afferens	8
Sorbitol	69	Vascular endothelial growth factor C	10
Soups	39	Vascular growth factor, endothelial (VEGF)	11
Sphingolipids	10		
Stamina	25	Vascular resistance	10, 12
Stamina training	25	Vasoconstriction	13
Stress, oxidative	14, 15, 23	Vasodilatation	12
Stroke	11, 12, 21	Vegetables	43
Substance, anti-oxidative	14	Vegetative nerve system	19
Sugar-protein molecules	19	Vibrancy of Food	22
Sunlight	18, 19, 22	Vital substances	23
Superoxide radical (O_2^-)	14	Vitamin A	14
System, anti-oxidative	21	Vitamin B12	22
System, dissipative	19	Vitamin C	14
		Vitamin E	14
Table, glycaemic charge	69		
Table, glycaemic index	69	Waves, standing	18
TAU proteins	15, 21	Weight reduction	24
Tertiary structure	15	White flour	12
Thermodynamics, first law of	17		

CENTRE FOR SCIENTIFIC NATURAL MEDICINE

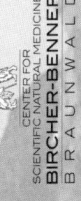

CENTER FOR SCIENTIFIC NATURAL MEDICINE
BIRCHER-BENNER
BRAUNWALD

People come to the Bircher-Benner Medical Centre from a large number of countries in search of healing.

Here, you will be valued as a unique person, listened to and understood. Here, humanity and dignity are important and the medicine is a noble undertaking.

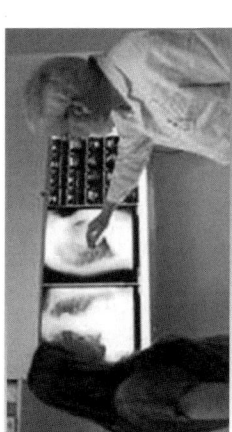

The search for the true causes of diseases is central to our work, as is the inclusion of your self-curative powers in the process of healing.

Centre for scientific natural medicine

Our fresh-vegetable diet will bring about a rapid change in your metabolism; natural regulative therapies take precedence where possible.

The atmosphere and the living tradition of the Bircher-Benner Centre, where novelty and modernity are combined with decades of experience, contribute to your healing.

The doctors and therapists will treat you personally and have all the facilities of a modern clinic at hand when needed.

The supplementation of traditional medicine by the regulative diagnosis and therapy of natural healing often permits a cure where the usual therapies have failed.

In the Medical Centre, you can relax and recover, and will experience the deep regeneration of your healing powers.

CENTRE BIRCHER-BENNER
CH-8784 Braunwald

Phone: +41 (0)21 801 60 04
Fax: +41 (0)55 643 16 93
info@bircher-benner.com
www.bircher-benner.com

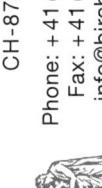

Indications: any internal diseases, migraine, tinnitus, neuralgia and other pain conditions, fibromyalgia, arthritis and arthrosis, collagenoses, liver, gallbladder and gastrointestinal diseases, metabolic diseases and diabetes, cardiovascular diseases, kidney and prostate diseases, women's diseases, allergies, skin diseases, convalescence, fatigue, depression and anxiety, menopausal, hormonal and weight problems.